GARBH SANSKAR

The Amazing Journey of Pregnancy

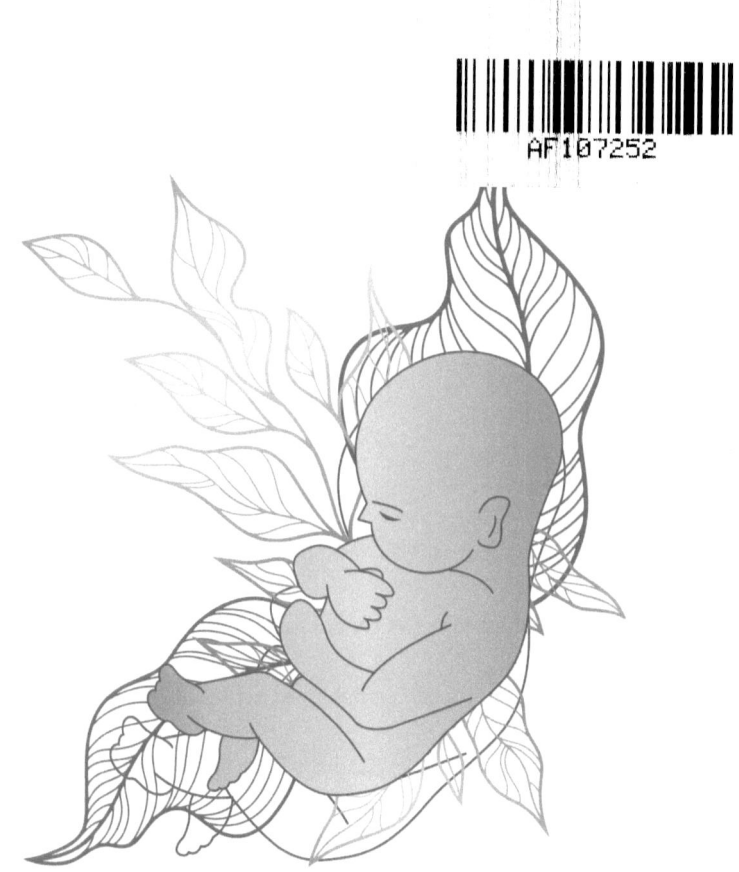

Profound Answers on the
Essence of Pregnancy and Childbirth

A Happy Thoughts Initiative

Garbh Sanskar
The Amazing Journey of Pregnancy
Profound Answers on the Essence of Pregnancy and Childbirth
By WOW Publishings Pvt. Ltd.

Copyright © WOW Publishings Pvt. Ltd.

All Rights Reserved 2024

ISBN : 978-93-90132-40-9

Published by WOW Publishings Pvt. Ltd., India

First edition published in June 2024

Printed and bound by Trinity Academy For Corporate Training Ltd, Pune

This book is based on the Hindi book titled -
Garbh Sanskar - Amazing Journey of Pregnancy

Copyright and publishing rights are vested exclusively with WOW Publishings Pvt. Ltd. This book is sold subject to the condition that it shall not by way of trade or otherwise, be lent, resold, hired out, or otherwise circulated without the publisher's prior written consent in any form of binding or cover other than that in which it is published and without a similar condition including this condition being imposed on the subsequent purchaser and without limiting the rights under copyright reserved above, no part of this publication may be reproduced, stored in or introduced into a retrieval system, or transmitted, in any form, or by any means, electronic, mechanical, photocopying, recording or otherwise, without the prior written permission of both the copyright owner and the above-mentioned publisher of this book. Any person who does any unauthorized act in relation to this publication may be liable to criminal prosecution and civil claims for damages.

Although the author and publisher have made every effort to ensure accuracy of content in this book, they hereby disclaim any liability to any party for any loss, damage, or disruption caused by errors or omissions, resulting from negligence, accident, or any other cause. Readers are advised to take full responsibility to exercise discretion in understanding and applying the content of this book.

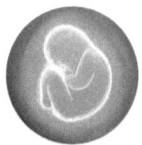

To every little one in the womb, about to enter this world,

Brimming with the immense potential of the Universe.

CONTENTS

Preface	7
PART I – Essential Planning for Pregnancy	
1. Instilling Values Before Pregnancy	12
2. Recognize Who is Coming	15
3. Introduction to Garbh Sanskar	20
4. Get Rid of Stress, Wear the Happy Hat	23
5. Impact of Environment on Pregnancy	27
6. The Mother's Emotions During Pregnancy	32
7. Three Attributes Governing Human Nature	37
8. The Foundation of a Balanced Life	42
9. See the Truth in Every Situation	47
10. Forgiveness to Purify Your Heart	51
11. Alignment with the Divine Will	56
12. Embrace Your Child's Uniqueness	59
13. The Feeling of Abundance	64
PART II – Instilling Higher Values in the Baby	
14. Center Your Focus to Instill Virtues	71
15. Conscious Conversation with the Baby	75
16. Impact of Gender Discrimination	79
17. Appreciation and Gratitude	82

| 18. Sow the Seeds of Benevolence | 87 |
| 19. Free the Child from Your Pain | 92 |

PART III – Right Conduct for a Pregnant Woman

20. Healthy Practices for the Day	99
21. Prenatal Nutrition and Wellness	104
22. Prenatal Clarity: Bridging Tradition and Truth	110
23. Hormones to Harmony	116
24. Essential Steps Before the Baby Arrives	120
25. Preparing Your Mind for Childbirth – 1	125
26. Preparing Your Mind for Childbirth – 2	130
27. The Multifaceted Essence of Motherhood – 1	135
28. The Multifaceted Essence of Motherhood – 2	139

PART IV – Answers on Closely Related Topics

29. Understanding Rebirth and Spiritual Evolution	147
30. Answers on Related Aspects	154
31. ResearchGate Survey and Findings	163
Appendix	166

Preface
The Heir of Higher Consciousness

When a seed sprouts and grows, many factors in its surroundings contribute to its blossoming, such as fertile soil, sunlight, air, and water. But the most crucial part is the plant itself, which bears the seed. If the plant is healthy and receives the right nourishment internally and externally, it leads to the beautiful sprouting and growth of the seed.

Similarly, many factors support the birth of a healthy, beautiful baby. They are a peaceful environment at home, harmonious relationships, economic stability, etc. But the most important factor is when the baby is in the womb, where the fetus grows, where the initial values and impressions of parental conditioning are inscribed in the child's psyche.

Earth is a school. We are born here to learn and evolve. As children grow, they go through accelerated learning when they begin school. But what if they get to learn some lessons at home? Wouldn't it be easier for them to understand it in school? In the same way, if the values and qualities one needs to develop in the school of earthly life are ingrained in the womb itself, wouldn't it be much easier for the child to blossom after birth? This process is called spiritual birthing, a method of educating the mind of an unborn baby in the womb and instilling higher values.

In a child's life journey, the mother plays the role of the first and most influential teacher. Her own life, mindset, and disposition lay the foundation of good moral values for her baby right from conception. History has witnessed many exceptional mothers who have instilled such values in children, helping them reach the pinnacle of excellence. For example, Prince Abhimanyu, from the Indian epic Mahabharata, received virtuous values from his mother, Subhadra; Mother Mary served as a medium to instill pure divine values in Jesus in her womb.

Every woman has the potential of giving birth to great personalities like Lord Rama, Lord Krishna, the Buddha, Lord Mahavira, Saint Kabir, Saint Tulsidas, Saint Meera, Jesus, Swami Vivekananda, and many more. Nothing is impossible in this world.

The development of the fetus' psyche largely depends on the emotions, thoughts, diet, and the environment around the expectant mother. Neurologists state that if a gestating mother is anxious, angry, or laments for a longer duration, it directly impacts the neurological development of the fetus. Research states that stress, anxiety, or depression in gestating mothers is associated with poor obstetric outcomes and demonstrates social, emotional, and behavioral challenges in their children.

A baby in the womb is like a lump of wet clay in the hands of a potter awaiting its final form. A potter gives the desired shape to the pliable clay, creating beautiful pots. Similarly, an expectant mother can help shape the baby into a divine, virtuous being by nourishing and molding it with the right diet, lifestyle, thoughts, and beliefs. Hence, she must first sculpt her own thoughts. She must work on removing the negative patterns and tendencies of her mind so that she is well-balanced and equipoised; so that she cultivates good habits within herself. The essence is that she must undergo this training when she is planning for a pregnancy or early in pregnancy so that it automatically permeates the unborn baby, laying a strong foundation for its growth and development.

This book is designed to help you with comprehensive guidance before conception and the knowledge required post-conception. The understanding made available through this book will also be imbibed by the baby through you. Embracing this understanding will bring love, joy, positivity, and a celebration of life in the family.

A deep understanding and all prenatal doubts are threaded in the form of questions and answers in this book. This book is a compilation of content that is largely based on guidance by Sirshree and also supported by research. You will receive straightforward, simple answers to your qualms centered on the prenatal evolution and divine conditioning of the baby. This is the age-old wisdom our ancestors passed on in the form of Garbh Sanskar. But this book provides that ancient wisdom in the present context. It is presented in a framework that makes it easier for today's women to understand and assimilate.

Over time, the knowledge imposed upon us in the form of mere rituals and traditions makes us skeptical, and we start questioning it. However, we quickly embrace the knowledge that resonates with our present-day needs. This same effort has been made in this book. Hence, everything that one needs to know and believe about sculpting the child's nature during pregnancy is compiled in this book so that one can assimilate it easily.

We hope this book makes you feel more connected with your baby in the womb and your pregnancy journey is blissful and happy.

PART I

Essential Planning for Pregnancy

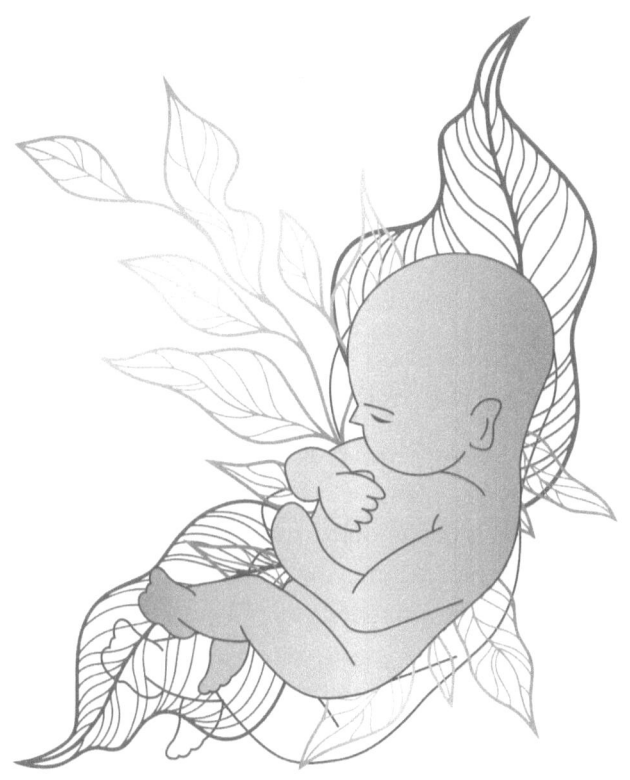

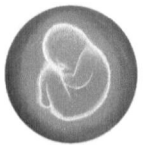

1
Instilling Values Before Pregnancy

Welcoming a child into this world is a joyful experience but it also carries a huge responsibility. A child is not a mere doll for the parents but rather represents the future of the world. Thus, it is the parent's responsibility to ensure the well-being of their child, physically and mentally. Doing so allows the child to enjoy life fully and actively contribute to building a healthy community.

Q: Is it necessary to plan for the betterment of the coming child?

A: Indeed, Yes. It is imperative for parents to plan and prepare for the baby much before conception and, as much as possible, avoid an accidental pregnancy. A baby is not an object that can be just brought home and kept like any other possession in the house. It is God's creation; it is an embodiment of Divine Consciousness. The child needs to be invoked with the same reverence and purity as one invokes God in worship. The parents should welcome the baby just as they would welcome a special guest.

It is the fundamental principle of nature: whatever we give our attention to, begins to come into our lives. So, the qualities that we focus on manifest in our lives. Hence, pray to God, "O God, let the child coming into our lives be blessed with divine qualities like love, courage, compassion, higher intelligence, perfect health, truthfulness, peace, simplicity, and innocence. May the baby's presence be as enchanting and beautiful as its innocent laughter. May the baby's arrival bring boundless joy, not just in our home but also to the world."

Q: Parents have many expectations from their prospective child; how can they be fulfilled?

A: Every parent wishes for an ideal child and wants to provide all the worldly pleasures to their beloved angel. They expect their child to possess divine qualities, be impeccable, just like the Higher Consciousness, and be a pious reflection of the Higher Consciousness itself. But pause for a moment; there is more that is needed.

Have you ever considered the kind of parents the child might expect? That subtle, pure being of Consciousness, who will come home as a baby, may also be making preparations.

Wherever that prospective child is, it also expects ideal parents for itself. The child also may be praying, "O God, may I get such parents who have a healthy body and mind and have divine qualities of love, joy, compassion, peace, and understanding. May they be full of tender love and care. May the house be filled with grace and harmony."

As parents, you too need to introspect whether you are a "Happy Mommy and Papa." Do you have a harmonious relationship as a couple, or do you squabble over minor issues? Do the differences of opinion persist? If yes, what would happen if the child refused to come into your life?

These questions are not to discourage you but to raise your awareness and make you understand that the preparations for the prospective child cannot be made half-heartedly. As parents, you have set your expectations about the kind of child you wish to have. But it is important that you, too, prepare for the kind of parent your child would expect. You also need to work on yourself even before conception to be able to welcome the baby wholeheartedly and happily.

In fact, a lot has been spoken about prenatal rituals, instilling values and habits in the baby after conception so that it becomes a good human being. However, only a few people talk about pre-conception practices that parents can learn. To learn and adopt these practices, parents should work hard on themselves and change their perspectives and habits. They need to be happy and peaceful to welcome a happy, cheerful baby.

Points for reflection

- The law of nature states, "What we focus on comes into our life." So, always focus on good qualities and positive thinking.
- Just as parents pray for the prospective child to be full of divine qualities, perfect health, and cheerfulness, the child also prays for the right parents. Hence, it is essential to adopt those qualities, which will become the foundation of a happy and peaceful world.
- Everyone is aware of the importance of instilling higher values and incorporating positive habits in the child after the baby's conception. However, it is important for the parents-to-be to consider the pre-conception practices that should be followed. They should reconsider their daily routine, behavioral patterns, and lifestyle while planning to conceive.

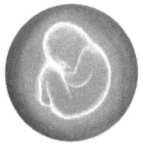

2
Recognize Who is Coming

Parents inadvertently often make the mistake of tagging the baby as "mine" upon the baby's birth or conception. Subsequently, they start building their expectations, "My child should be beautiful, healthy, smart, and intelligent. My child should be obedient, adhere to my instructions, and follow my routine of sleep, waking up, eating, drinking, and so forth."

If a baby is born with some health challenges or displays habits and behavior that are different from the parents', the parents find it difficult to accept them entirely. Such parents remain unhappy throughout their lives. They always try to mold their child as they wish, although such efforts prove futile.

Q: After all, my child will be mine; what is wrong with keeping expectations?

A: Before understanding the answer to this question, it is important to reflect on some profound questions, like,

- Who is this being that is coming?
- Why is that being coming into your life?
- Why only in your life and not anyone else's?
- What is your relationship with that being?
- What right do you have on that being?
- Why are you so eager to instill values and habits in that being?

If parents understand these aspects even before the arrival of the baby, their parental life can be fulfilling; otherwise, they will invite sorrow into their lives. As a result, they will make their children sad and miserable.

Let's understand the repercussions of expectations with the help of an example from the life of the Buddha. King Shuddhodhana was an ambitious king and aspired for his son, Prince Siddhartha, to become a great emperor. But Siddhartha had a different divine plan. His thinking and behavior contradicted his father's ambitious desires. King Shuddhodhana could not accept this. He tried his best to distract Siddhartha from the path of Truth. But we all know what happened eventually. Siddhartha quietly left his kingdom in pursuit of the Truth. As a result, the king and the royal family had to endure sorrow while Siddhartha, too, struggled through his journey to enlightenment.

Wouldn't it have been beneficial if Siddhartha's father refrained from tagging Siddhartha as "my son." If he had wholeheartedly accepted Siddhartha's divine plan, considering it his duty to align with the Creator's divine plan, if he had supported Siddhartha by providing him with the necessary resources to fulfill his divine purpose, Siddhartha's journey would have been less arduous. He wouldn't have had to resort to such a drastic step of leaving his kingdom.

Let us consider another example of Saint Tulsidas. His father had abandoned him at birth because he believed that being born in *Moola Nakshatra*, an inauspicious configuration according to Vedic astrology, would be troublesome for the parents. However, we all know how Saint Tulsidas lived as a devout saint. He expressed his devotion through divine poetry and spiritual literature. However, he endured a painful childhood as he did not meet his father's expectations. Had his father known about the great saint embodied in his child, he wouldn't have cast him away.

Parents keep expecting from their children based on what seems right from their own standpoint and understanding. However, their viewpoint and understanding need not always align with the child's divine plan. It is important for parents to gain this understanding even before conception.

With this, they can possibly avoid the ill effects of their wrong beliefs or perspectives on the innocent baby.

These days, many parents decide the profession or career path their prospective child should pursue even before the baby is born! They prefix whether the child should become a doctor, engineer, chartered accountant, or scientist. However, with the example from Siddhartha's life, we have understood that the child may have a different divine purpose.

Let us now understand the answers to the questions asked initially.

- The baby coming into your household is not just a physical entity formed by the union of a man and a woman but, more importantly, a pure being, an expression of Higher Consciousness.
- The child is not your personal property but is independent and has his or her own inherent nature, values, experiences, memories, and deeds. The child has reasons and a divine plan for being born.
- The child is not part of your personal plan; rather, you are a part of the Creator's divine plan for the child.
- The parents may feel that they have conceived, but the truth is that the Higher Consciousness, Source, God, or Self, whatever name you wish to call it, has chosen this womb to be conceived.
- Every living being takes birth on Earth for a purpose of their own. It could be some preordained divine manifestation or an opportunity to break free of karmic bondages. They come to play their part on this world's stage, which nature has determined for them, not merely to fulfill the parents' expectations.
- Parents have a similar role with their children as gardeners have with their garden. The gardener takes care of the garden to the best of his or her ability, leaving the rest to God. The

gardener is responsible for watering the plants, providing the right fertilizer, nourishing them, and loving them. But it is up to nature how many flowers will bloom, how many fruits they will bear, and how long they will survive. Similarly, parents, too, have to take care of their children to the best of their abilities, acknowledging that the outcomes are beyond their control and determined by nature.

- The parent's duty towards the prospective child is to give it a conducive environment and selfless love to blossom and express their fullest potential. It is their responsibility to support the child completely and not bind them in attachment and expectations. Parents who have unconditionally supported their children have brought wonders into their children's earthly life.

This is a unique and revolutionary outlook toward children. Parents need to contemplate and see their children and themselves with this new perspective. Reflect on your parents' expectations of you. Did they ever seem like bondage or restrictions to you? Would you like to impose the same restrictions on your children?

When you accept the prospective child as an independent expression of the divine being, your prayers, thoughts, feelings, and expectations will change. This new approach will change the lives of both – the parents and the child.

Q: How will this happen?

A: With this understanding, your prayers will shift from personal to impersonal. For example, when someone who lacks this understanding prays for their prospective child's qualities like love, courage, compassion, intelligence, and perfect health, they will say, "May our child demonstrate the best qualities." But after gaining this new understanding, their prayer will change. They will say, "Let the child that chooses our house be blessed with divine qualities," i.e., they wish for the divine qualities in the child not for their own sake but for the divine expression through the child.

With this new perspective, the prayer would be, "O God, give us the right understanding, with which we can take care of the precious gift who will grace our house. Give us the strength to fully support the divine being and provide a favorable and healthy life. Help us give a healthy environment where the pure being can easily fulfill their divine plan, which you have chosen for them."

As a result, decisions made for children with this new understanding will be appropriate as they transcend selfishness. If this happens, the child will become sacred and virtuous, capable of expressing a higher way of life to the fullest.

Points for reflection

- Give a new positive direction to the mind so that it lets go of the old ways of confusing thinking patterns of the mind and focuses on creating a new vision of the future.
- Avoid tagging the baby as "my child" right from pregnancy and be instrumental in inviting and receiving divine qualities for the child.
- The pure being growing in the womb is not merely a physical body but an embodiment of Higher Consciousness. Hence, it is essential to catalyze the child's growth and development according to the child's divine plan.
- Self or consciousness itself chooses the womb through which it wishes to incarnate. Hence, parents have only as much right over the child as a gardener would have over his or her garden.

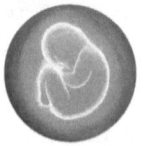

3
Introduction to Garbh Sanskar

In digital language, we can call our brain a hard disk that stores data. The hard disk of a baby in the womb is connected to the mother's brain. As a result, the mother's thoughts, feelings, perspective of life, behavioral traits, etc., get etched in the unborn baby's brain. During pregnancy, the mother experiences a lot of mood swings that create imprints, also known as *Sanskar* or impressions, in the unborn baby's mind. Hence, despite being genetically identical, siblings can be different as the mother's mood and emotional state during each pregnancy differ.

Q: How was the word Garbh Sanskar coined? What does it mean?

A: *Garbh Sanskar* is a Sanskrit term, where *Garbh* means womb and *Sanskar* means impressions. Sanskar also means purification, instilling the seeds of higher values at the right time to keep oneself pure and virtuous.

Our qualities, behavioral traits, and inclinations together form our nature. When someone is taught something new that they imbibe into their life, they are said to receive the sanskar. Since ancient times, passing higher values to the next generation as sanskar has always been a part of the Indian tradition.

Sanskar also means sacrament or holy rite, performed to mark the commencement of a new phase of human life. The journey of human development from birth to death is divided into 16 sacraments. As one progresses in life, we need to embrace these 16 sanskars, or sacraments, that are traditionally marked by rites performed at various milestones in the passage of life. This is to ensure that we progress in all areas of life holistically. All these sacraments were religiously practiced in olden times.

Of these 16 sacraments, the first sacrament centers around conception. This sanskar elucidates the right understanding of conception and provides guidance about the intricacies of the birthing process during the nine-month gestation period. As life unfolds, embracing each sacrament, we culminate this journey with the last or concluding sanskar of the funeral. The consciousness that enters this world with the conception sacrament exits this world with the funeral sacrament and continues its further journey.

Q: How can one conceive with the right understanding and knowledge of Garbh Sanskar?

A: Conceiving is a part of Garbh Sanskar. It is a pious deed and can also be referred to as Spiritual birthing. It should not be contaminated with lust. With conception, you are inviting an embodiment of pure consciousness into this world. The body is going to serve this sacred cause. Hence, your thoughts and feelings during conception need to be untainted to welcome a pure being. The generator of the world is entrusting you with the divine task of ushering a new generation into this world. Hence, this must be considered a divine endeavor that demands a deep sense of responsibility.

Let us understand the purpose of Garbh Sanskar in simple words, with the help of an example. When we board a bus, we focus on getting the most comfortable and best among the available seats. Similarly, when a pure being chooses a womb, it also seeks a family, a womb, which would make its journey of life happy and purposeful and help in fulfilling its divine purpose of life on Earth.

The birth of the baby should not be a sudden accidental event; it should be preplanned. The husband and wife need to be completely prepared mentally and physically. This is because, after conception, the physical health and mental well-being of the parents have the most impact on the baby. They need to make amendments to their routine habits, including their thinking, eating, conversing, reading, and so on, well before pregnancy. They need to think positively, and if there is any difference of opinion between the husband and wife, it should be settled before conception. Any stress during pregnancy can adversely affect the child's mental and physical growth.

It is also essential to have a happy, peaceful, healthy, and harmonious environment instead of stress, worry, and diseases. Both parents should be able to care for the prospective child in every way and be mentally prepared for it.

Points for reflection

- In the primary sense, sacrament, or sanskar, is developing the right qualities at the right time by maintaining one's purity.
- There are 16 sanskars or sacraments that a human being traverses in the journey of life from birth to death. The first one is that of conception or the Garbh Sanskar.
- For the arrival of a pure being, the thoughts and feelings of the parents need to be pure at conception.

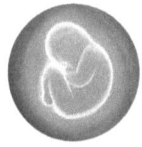

4

Get Rid of Stress, Wear the Happy Hat

"Let go of the past and focus in the present." We all might have heard this sentence at some point in life. This phrase can work like a mantra. It can free us from the bondage of past mistakes and help us develop clarity on the way ahead. Otherwise, we tend to be lost in the fog of the burden of the past.

Q: What if the pregnancy is accidental and not pre-planned? If the husband and wife are not mentally prepared for this, will it be detrimental for the child-to-be?

A: We are always delighted when we gain a new and positive understanding. But there's another downside to it: we feel fearful or regretful.

We fear whether we will be able to apply the understanding we are gaining properly. We regret, "Alas! It would have been better if I had learned these truths earlier. Life would have been way easier!" We feel guilty thinking, "I don't know how many mistakes I have committed in ignorance."

The same applies to the journey of pregnancy. Pregnancy should be planned with complete preparation. One needs to be physically, mentally, and emotionally prepared and invoke the new being with auspicious prayers and a sacred feeling. But while this is true, it is never too late to begin. This perspective will help in raising awareness and gaining knowledge. With this new understanding of Garbh Sanskar, life can be illuminated by the radiant sun of knowledge. Why worry about the past? Let's understand this with the help of a story.

A cloth merchant would carry clothes on horseback to sell them in the market. He earned a lot of money by selling clothes and kept the coins in a bag. It so happened that rats had gnawed at his bag, boring a hole in it. On his way back, the coins began to spill out one by one. Every evening, when he would count the coins, he noticed that the count had reduced. He kept lamenting the loss. He failed to understand that he could save the rest of his coins by sealing that hole. Gradually, all the coins fell off the bag.

Now, what would you tell this cloth merchant, who was mourning over what was lost? He never thought about what could still be saved or salvaged, nor did he try to prevent further loss. Whatever has happened in the past is over; worrying about it serves no purpose. It is wise to secure what is left.

Drawing parallels to the story, a prospective mother needs to understand that even if two or three months of pregnancy have passed, the journey is yet to come to term. Later, even when the child is born, you have the entire life to make changes or work on instilling the right values in your child. The understanding you gain about Garbh Sanskar through this book will stay with you forever. These practices of spiritual birthing have been prevalent in the past, are followed today, and will continue to be practiced even in the future, even after the delivery of the baby. Hence, instead of mourning over the missed opportunity, it is wiser to start working on it now. Now is the best time to start. As rightly said, it is never too late to begin. So start applying the lessons learned hereon and bring transformation in your life and your baby's life, too.

While you understand the importance of instilling higher values, here is another important question that needs to be addressed: Who is teaching whom?

Parents often think, "We will teach our child how to become a better person," but the reality is that the child is coming to teach you how to live. Your child is here to help you change your perspective toward life and refine the way you lead life. Parents feel, "By learning about Garbh

Sanskar, we will instill divine qualities in the baby." But the divine qualities are already a part of the Creator's divine creation, your baby. The child is a goldmine of divine attributes. The prospective child is coming to awaken divine qualities in you. It is a medium to help you nurture divine qualities like unconditional love, patience, joy, peace, forgiveness, and goodwill so that you live your life to the fullest.

Q: How do we compensate for the time lost by not preparing beforehand? How can we be assured and stay calm and relaxed?

A: The simplest and direct answer to this question is wearing a Happy Hat, i.e., an attitude of happiness. This Hat is not found in any store but is already within us. One must wear it at all times. When we wear this Hat, we put aside all the guilt and worries about the future and surrender ourselves to nature. We affirm to nature, "Thy will is my will," which means whatever nature wishes for me is my wish, too; I align with what nature desires for me.

The right method of wearing the Happy Hat is by surrendering yourself to nature and staying relaxed in full faith. You perform your duties with an attitude of acceptance by rejoicing in the feeling that the One who is taking care of everyone in the world is taking care of your baby, too.

So, do not regret that time has passed and you have lost the opportunity. Do not be stressed or overwhelmed about teaching the child something or learning it yourself. Let go of all fears and negativity around pregnancy. Just live in the present moment, be in the free flow of nature, and perform all your actions with purity to the extent possible. Whatever nature wants to get done through you will be done. You need to remain happy in the present moment. This is the key to giving the best environment to the child. If this happens, all the family members, parents, and the child will be happy.

Points for reflection

- Don't worry if you are late in understanding the principles of conception and Garbh Sanskar. You can still instill divine virtues and higher values in the child.

- The prospective child is coming to awaken divine qualities within you.
- Wear your Happy Hat at all times; the Hat of happiness is within you. Do not hold onto guilt or regret over past mistakes, and do not worry about the future. Surrender to nature and affirm, "Thy will is my will; whatever you wish is my wish."

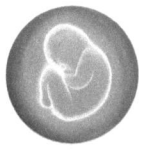

5
Impact of Environment on Pregnancy

Although the baby grows in the mother's womb, it is also influenced by the surroundings that shape its physical and mental development. This is like a sapling that receives nourishment not just from the soil through its roots but also from external elements like sunlight, air, and water to support its growth. If one understands this science, they will support the baby's physical and mental development.

Q: It is said that the baby growing in the womb is like a blank canvas; any values or mental impressions can be inscribed on it. Along with this, it is also said that the baby brings along tendencies from its previous lives. What is the reality?

A: We all have used a diary or notebook to write. If we carefully observe the blank pages of the diary, we can see the subtle impression of the text written on its previous page. Also, light impressions of what is written on pages that precede the previous page can also be seen. Sometimes, these impressions are so strong that we can easily read them without registering them in ink.

Similarly, we can say that the baby has some impressions from memories that are planted into it. These memories play a vital role in determining the baby's behavioral traits, qualities, and instincts. Further, when the baby is conceived in the mother's womb, new impressions are fed into its psyche. Let us understand this in detail.

The first, or the direct method, that creates impressions is genetics, heredity. A child inherits some qualities and traits through the genes of its parents and ancestors. These qualities could be – physical, mental, or emotional. These genetic qualities are often visible in the child's appearance or behavior. Along with qualities and behavioral traits, a child can also inherit physical disorders and emotional conditions.

There is also a second method called epigenetics. Epigenetics is a field of modern science that deals with the influences created through the surrounding environment. From ancient times, Indian culture has believed that the child is not only shaped genetically but through its surroundings as well. The family, society, and surroundings in which the child grows, play an important role in influencing its development.

Our ancestors were well aware of the epigenetic effects on the baby. Hence, along with the physical, mental, and emotional well-being of the parents, they also believed in maintaining purity in the surroundings as a whole. They further emphasized maintaining purity and sanity at the level of thought. They strongly believed that everything around the womb, both positive and negative, impacts the baby. Hence, maintaining sanity in the environment, especially around the pregnant mother, was given special attention. Similar efforts were made by imparting higher wisdom through Garbh Sanskar, the divine birthing, to proliferate positive epigenetic impact and eliminate the negative.

In the last few years, this old tradition has mostly been overlooked. However, as awareness is increasing, people are now re-adopting the divine birthing sacraments. After ample research, even medical science has accepted that the baby growing in the womb is as conscious and aware as the baby after birth. The baby's senses and emotions have already started functioning while it is still in the womb. It can hear, feel, and perceive inputs. The baby continuously records and stores information it receives through its mother and the surrounding environment in its memory. Its database gets prepared in the womb itself.

Indian mythology is replete with examples of children who received divine impressions in their mother's womb. One such example is Prince Abhimanyu, the son of the Pandava Prince Arjuna, from the Indian epic,

Mahabharata. He learned how to enter the *Chakravyuh*, a maze-like battle formation used in warfare during those days, while he was still in the womb. It is the most apt example of the baby gaining knowledge or information in the womb. The formation of a child's personality, conduct, and behavioral traits begins here.

In fact, the thoughts and behavior of two siblings are different. Because their formation is influenced not just by the mother's state of mind but also by many other surrounding or external factors. The mother may have lived in a different environment during one pregnancy and a completely different one during the other. The mother's state of mind during both pregnancies would be different, directly or indirectly affecting the baby.

Another good example from the Indian scriptures is the life of Prahlad, an ardent devotee of Lord Vishnu. His father, Hiranyakashyap, was the demon clan's king and possessed a demonic nature. He was a staunch opponent of Lord Vishnu.

Once, the deities and demons had a war in which they defeated Hiranyakashyap. They wanted to destroy all the demons. Hiranyakashyap's wife was pregnant then. Sage Narada, another ardent disciple of Lord Vishnu, offered her shelter in his hermitage to safeguard her during her pregnancy. Now, this was a complete change in the external environment for the baby in the womb. Earlier, she lived amidst demons possessing violent tendencies. Now, she and the baby growing in her womb were surrounded by supreme peace and devotion, listening to the sacred chantings of Lord Vishu.

The seeds of devotion to Lord Vishnu were automatically sown while Prahlad was still in his mother's womb and sprouted in his life later. Prahlad grew up to become a firm devotee of Lord Vishnu and chanted "Narayan… Narayan…" all day. This would not have been possible if his mother's surroundings had not changed. Although it is possible that she possessed devotional memories, those memories were awakened only after receiving a favorable environment like Sage Narada's Ashram.

Q: If the surroundings influence the baby in the womb, why are all the rules and regulations made only for the mother? Why is only she considered responsible for instilling values and receiving sacraments for the child?

A: There are three reasons for this. The first reason is ignorance. People believe that the mother alone influences the child; hence, she is advised to follow all kinds of rules, attend spiritual discourses or sacred gatherings, etc.

The second reason is that it is difficult to improve oneself, as it takes a lot of hard work. Thus, the rest of the family entrusts all the responsibility to the mother.

The third and most important reason is if the baby is to be considered as a blank page, then the mother is the filled-in page just above that blank page. The mother is the closest to the child and has the greatest influence on the baby. The baby's subconscious mind is connected to that of the mother. Not only the food she eats but her thoughts and emotions also impact the baby directly. The father comes next after the mother in the degree of influence. His emotions and energy also have a profound impact on the child. In this way, every person in the mother's vicinity has some impact on the child.

As the impressions created by the mother's state of mind on the baby are more profound, she has been entrusted with the responsibility of receiving the Garbh Sanskar or the values of divine pregnancy. Only a mother has the power to protect the baby from being influenced by adverse situations. She can erase the impact of negative thoughts from the environment with her positive thoughts, thus ring fencing the child's psyche during this delicate period.

But it's important to understand that this power does not come all at once. It does not happen that all of a sudden, one day, the woman realizes she is pregnant and starts thinking positively, stops worrying, and stays happy. These habits of positive thinking and maintaining emotional fortitude should be a part of her nature. It is foolish to dig a well when one is thirsty. One needs to arrange for water long before feeling thirsty. It is important to work on oneself and adopt a positive, healthy, happy lifestyle long before conception.

The mother's inner world, i.e., her thoughts, feelings, and emotions, undoubtedly impact the child more than the physical environment. Therefore, one needs to primarily work on internal purification while also creating a conducive environment, and this needs to be done by the parents and all the family members together.

Points for reflection

- A baby growing in the womb is as conscious as a baby after birth. Its senses and emotions are active in the womb itself. It can hear and feel the words, thoughts, and feelings entertained by the parents. Hence, parents should be aware of and absorb only positive inputs from the surrounding environment.
- The subconscious mind of the baby is connected to the subconscious mind of the mother. She is closest to the baby and has the greatest influence on the baby. Hence, the mother is entrusted with the responsibility of receiving divine pregnancy sacraments. She has the power to stop the negative influences from the surroundings with positive thoughts and instill the right values in the baby.

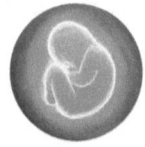

6

The Mother's Emotions During Pregnancy

We all know how our whimsical mind works and the cards it plays, making the graph of life go up and down like a rollercoaster. The sooner we understand the tricks of the mind, the faster we can stabilize this graph. This acrobatic mind plays a vital role in a pregnant lady's birthing journey. Let's take a look at it.

Life is a journey; each day is a small part of this big journey. Each day, we undergo an array of emotions, sometimes high and sometimes low. Have we considered pausing for a moment just to understand how often the mind changes its graph? Especially on the lower side. How often does one feel hurt? What makes them feel disappointed? When do the emotions turn negative? Which habits and attitudes compel them to think in a particular manner?

These negative feelings or emotions adversely affect our physical and mental health. Only by resolving these with the right understanding can we curb this negativity to heal our bodies. As we progress through this healing journey, we can instill the right values and principles in the baby. Hence, along with the expectant mother, other family members should also consider contemplating the above questions.

Q: How do the mother's emotions affect the baby?

A: The process of instilling the right seeds in the baby, i.e., the right thinking, qualities, habits, etc., can start right after conception. Most of the programming of the child's psyche happens in the womb through the expectant mother's feelings, thought patterns, and emotions. Simply put, a child enters the world as a reflection of the mother's emotions. For example, before baking the brick in the furnace, a name or design is imprinted on it with a stamp. When the brick is baked in the furnace, the design gets permanently engraved on it. In the same way, the mother's feelings also get etched on the child's heart and brain forever. It stays with the child even after birth. Hence, the mother needs to be vigilant and continuously work on her feelings, thoughts, and emotions, as they are the most important aspects during the pregnancy journey.

Whatever a woman receives through her five senses affects her body. The kind of food she eats will impact her health. What she hears, the scenes she sees, and her experiences affect her mind, body, and intellect. In turn, everything she does will also create the same impressions on the baby in the womb as well, just like the analogy of the impressions on the paper. Whatever you write on a sheet of paper is imprinted on the sheet below it. In the same way, everything that the mother holds in her mind, such as thoughts and emotions, gets etched as tendencies and behavioral patterns in the baby growing inside the womb. Hence, the sacraments given during the birthing process become crucial in shaping the child's personality.

In India, as soon as a lady conceives, the elders in her house, friends, and relatives start advising her on various things. They advise her to stay happy and cheerful, avoid negative thinking, take care of her diet, and always harbor positive and good thoughts. She is also advised to read holy scriptures like the Ramayana, Bhagavad Gita, Quran, Bible, Guru Granth Sahib, etc., and attend spiritual discourses or sacred gatherings.

She takes care of everything she is advised to, from altering her eating habits to inculcating the habit of good reading, attending spiritual discourses, etc. But all this is physical. She has no control over her thoughts and feelings. She cannot be forced to sit like a pleasing child. Her thoughts and emotions continue to run amok.

For example, while listening to a spiritual discourse, she may recollect a hurtful incident of the past that may trigger a chain of negative thoughts or feelings of ill-will towards a relative with whom she does not perhaps share a good bond. When a person forcibly tries to think positively, the negativity within comes out even more forcefully. That is why the negativity within tends to surface most prominently during meditation or devotional practices. Our feelings and thoughts change only when we gain the right understanding and wisdom, and not by forceful abidance to someone's advice.

Q: What is that understanding which, when received, can change our negative feelings to positive?

A: To attain that understanding, you must reflect on your deep-rooted thinking patterns, habits, and tendencies that enslave you. These patterns and tendencies can manifest as reactions to external triggers like social interactions and even to internal triggers such as biased interpretations and thoughts about the past or the future.

Q: Can you explain these patterns or tendencies in detail?

A: Every human being is programmed to think and react in a particular manner. Unknowingly, they think and respond the same way each time. It is called behavioral pattern. Some people quickly get angry at others' unacceptable behavior or carelessness. They think, how can someone be so stupid or do such stupid things? At work, they cannot tolerate the attitudes of their co-workers. The same happens at home as well. Such people, be it at home or the workplace, often remain unhappy.

People with this disposition experience frustration when work remains unfinished or is not completed on time. They always find one or the other flaw in others. They just need an excuse to get angry. They can be categorized as individuals with a perfectionist pattern.

Some people are always anchored in fear of lack. They are always anxious about the sustainability of their finances, happiness, and relationships. They fear it might not last. They are always worried about the future and burdened with insecurities. These people are consumed by fear and anxiety.

Some individuals are always unhappy. They keep reminiscing about old incidents and are unwilling to let go of past incidents when someone responded rudely, misbehaved, or ignored them. As these incidents are deep-rooted in their mind, they find it challenging to forgive people and often feel dejected. They have a desolation pattern.

Some people resist change; they cannot accept it easily. They are anxious and refrain from handling change in life. They feel that it will create a big stir in their life. They prefer living in their comfort zone. Imagine if a lady with this pattern conceives; what would her condition be like? She will have to undergo a hundred changes during her prenatal and post-natal period. How will she handle them?

Q: It seems challenging to navigate and break free from these patterns, isn't it?

A: No, it is not as challenging as it seems. If you are ready to observe, accept, and embrace your shortcomings, it is the first step to break free from these tendencies. Further, you just need the right understanding.

Q: What understanding?

A: Human beings are mainly governed by three basic dispositions. These are *Tamas* (Lethargy), *Rajas* (Hyperactivity) and *Sattva* (Virtuousness). It is crucial to understand these three dispositions. As soon as one understands these dispositions, one will realize why one harnesses a particular set of thoughts and reacts in a particular manner. Then, their outlook toward people will also change.

We will discuss these dispositions in the next chapter.

Points for reflection
- The mother's feelings are imprinted in the baby's heart and brain forever, which remains with it even after birth. Hence, women, especially when pregnant, are advised to take care of their diet, thoughts, and emotions and read sacred books.

- Man is a slave of habits and tendencies that run deep. Understanding these tendencies can help in navigating through them. This will help in changing their outlook toward people.

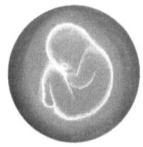

7
Three Attributes Governing Human Nature

How often have you observed and mused over people's behavior, "How can they do this? How can they be so silly? If I were in their place, I wouldn't have done this; I would have done that…"

Every person harbors such thoughts for others. And these questions always remain unanswered. Let us try to understand them through some ensuing questions and answers.

Q. What is human beings' inherent programming or nature that influences their behavior and controls their thoughts?

A. The Bhagavad Gita describes human nature as *Triguni Prakriti*, the threefold nature. This prakriti (nature) governs the behavioral traits, thoughts, intelligence, feelings, and habits of every human being.

Every aspiring parent envisions their future child to be an ideal child – one who excels in every task, is obedient, energetic, disciplined, mature, and devoid of anger and carelessness. They wish that the child be blessed with the ability to make the right decisions and grow up as a good human being, bringing acclaim to them. They also aspire that their child will contribute to the well-being of the family and the society. However, it is not necessary that the child would embody all these qualities, and these aspirations would materialize.

Pause for a moment and think: Your parents might have also had such expectations and prayers for you. Introspect honestly and ask yourself whether you have fully lived up to their expectations. Were you their ideal child?

If you weren't, there is no need to feel bad about it. The truth is that a person cannot always align their behavior according to others' expectations. They act or behave according to their inherent nature. As mentioned earlier, these behavioral traits are determined by their intrinsic nature, referred to as the Triguni Prakriti, which comprises three *gunas* or attributes. These three gunas are Tamas, Rajas, and Sattva: Lethargy, Hyperactivity, and Virtuousness. The relative proportion of these three attributes governs every individual.

In every individual, any one of these attributes is dominant, while the other two remain less dominant. This dominant guna influences their thinking pattern, intellectual faculty, feelings, and actions. By understanding these three attributes, one gains insights into why people behave as they do.

Q: Our present nature is shaped by the upbringing we have received; what difference will it make now? We have to instill the pregnancy sacraments in the baby, don't we?

A. Sacraments are not mere preaching. They are more than just spoken words. They are shaped and radiated by the parent's behavior, thoughts, feelings, and energy. The child's subconscious mind learns and absorbs the parent's conduct. Hence, isn't it imperative that the parents start practicing them first?

Q: Yes, I agree. So then, can you briefly explain these attributes and how they work?

A. Sure. Let's begin with Tamas. The fundamental nature of Tamas, denoting lethargy or sloth, is hidden in the name itself. Tama means darkness, which signifies ignorance, sorrow, and laziness. Tamas symbolizes physical inactivity. People with dominant Tamas guna, referred to as *Tamoguni* or people with *Tamasic* disposition, are habitually lazy, often oversleep, and tend to procrastinate. They do not want to exert themselves with any taxing work and often delay or postpone their work, regardless of the number of excuses they need to make or losses they might incur. Lethargy dominates their intellect as well. They are unable to make the right decisions. They primarily focus on the brief moments of pleasure and lack a visionary outlook or foresight. They seldom succeed, and even when they do, they cannot sustain the success for long. Rather than taking ownership, Tamasic people attribute their flaws and failures to people around them or to their perceived lack of fortune.

Q. How does Tamas affect a prospective mother?

A. Excess Tamas is harmful to both the pregnant mother and the baby. She finds excuses to oversleep and delays activity, primarily driven by reluctance and sometimes under the pretext of nausea. Surely, nausea can take its toll during the period of pregnancy, but one should be honest to oneself and introspect whether it is genuinely debilitating or being exaggerated to avoid activity. Tamoguni people rest excessively, leading to excess weight gain that shells their enthusiasm.

Q: And this excess weight gain invites other problems as well. In that case, Rajas would be another extreme. What are the indicators of Rajas?

A. Rajas indicates hyperactivity, a fundamental trait that exists in all to some extent. Rajas awakens desires and ambitions, propelling the individual to pursue them feverishly. People with a *Rajasic* nature find it challenging to attain calmness. Their mantra is "What next?" or "What do I do now?" Having multiple tasks on hand, no sooner than one task is accomplished, their mind is already racing toward restlessly completing the next task in a row.

Imagine the effect of such hyperactivity on a pregnant woman's health. She will always feel exhausted due to excessive activity. It will be a challenge for her to rest, as she will always be agitated to accomplish something or the other. Her mind will be racing ahead, filled with future anxiety. This anxiety can harm her and the baby's health.

This trait is often evident in children who can never sit peacefully. They are always on the run, onto some mischief or the other, running here, jumping there. Their sleep duration is significantly less than their peers.

Q: How is Sattva different from Rajas and Tamas?

A. A person with Sattvic nature captivates the hearts compared to Rajas and Tamas. Sattva includes virtues such as peace, equanimity, purity, wisdom, good character, conduct, service, and compassion. People with dominant Sattva never succumb to lethargy in their pursuits, nor do they rush feverishly through their tasks. Their approach to work is prompt with the right precision and poise. They think beyond personal interests and are mindful of their benevolent deeds.

The predominance of Sattva in a pregnant woman is very beneficial, but she must also be careful not to overdo it. For example, punctuality is a virtue. Adhering to a good routine, like sleeping and waking up on time, exercising regularly, and maintaining healthy eating habits, helps maintain a good balance. It is beneficial for the mother's mental and physical health.

But, while this is a blessing, she should be mindful that this blessing can become a curse. While maintaining a balanced lifestyle, she should be willing to embrace flexibility and imperfections in her routine, people, and surroundings. She needs to be watchful about the disturbance her mind can create while experiencing unpredictable changes that appear in the pregnancy journey.

Thus, being virtuous is the best attribute, a blessing one can aim at. People with Sattvic nature are inherently balanced, but they must allow and accommodate imperfections in people or their environment.

Points for reflection

- Human nature comprises three gunas or attributes. Our aim should be to recognize our dominant guna, enhance good attributes, and minimize the demerits.
- People cannot align their behavior according to others' expectations; they act according to their inherent nature.
- Children absorb values by observing their parent's conduct, thoughts, feelings, and the energy they radiate. Values cannot be imparted through mere words.

- Everyone exhibits Rajas in varying degrees, which is important, but an excess of anything is harmful, and so is hyperactivity.
- Sattva is better than Rajas and Tamas. It is a blessing that needs to be developed without making it a curse.

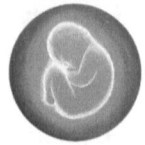

8
The Foundation of a Balanced Life

Q: Given that every attribute has some pros and cons, what state should we aim for?

A: We all know the secret recipe for delicious food – blending all the ingredients and spices in the right proportion in the right manner and cooking it for the required time. An excess or lack of any ingredient while cooking can affect its flavor, ruining its taste. The same applies to life, too!

To be happy, healthy, prosperous, peaceful, and creative, it is necessary to balance all three gunas. Balance implies just what is required, neither more nor less. Any quality in excess or deficiency can be harmful. The crux of a successful life is an apt and balanced expression of these three attributes devoid of attachment to any particular attribute.

If these three attributes, Sattva, Rajas, and Tamas, are balanced in a child right from the beginning, their life will be smooth, simple, and successful. But this is possible only when the parents lead their lives, balancing these three attributes. Hence, they need to understand and start working on balancing these gunas before the baby is conceived. This is important as it deeply impacts the baby in the womb.

For example, if the mother is tamasic in nature, she is lethargic, dull, and lazy; the child will also absorb these traits. On the other hand, children of virtuous parents inherit virtuousness right from childhood. A pregnant woman needs to identify her dominant guna and work on balancing the rest. By doing this, she can gradually attain a state where she can leverage all these attributes and eventually avoid the potential harm that any dominant attribute can cause.

Q: What can be done to attain this state?

A: The easiest way is to log your 24-hour routine. List everything you do, including the hours you sleep, work, rest, time spent on entertainment, etc. Assess the worth of your tasks. Reflect on your feelings while doing those tasks. Record the time spent on non-productive activities like gossiping or back-biting others. How much time is spent on entertainment such as the TV, the non-essential use of the mobile, Internet surfing, and social media?

Do you allocate some time in the day to render some service or selfless activity for others' welfare? It could be anything from helping your neighbor or colleague at the office to offering support to those in need, donating, praying selflessly for others, etc.

Now, observe what kind of activities dominate your daily routine. Which attribute influences your actions the most – Sattva, Rajas, or Tamas?

Do you sleep more than necessary or avoid work in favor of rest? Is your mind succumbing to lethargy? Are you wasting undue time on entertainment? All this stems from excessive laziness. You will have to address these issues and work on overcoming them. For example, you can give simple instructions to your body, "Rest at the time of rest, but work when it is time to work." Even after sufficient rest, if the body is reluctant to leave the bed, it must be roused with the right understanding. Allot specific time to watch TV, the mobile, or any entertainment; however, restrict it as far as possible. Once the time is up, close and move away. If the mind wanders into unnecessary thoughts and chatters, bring it back with awareness.

Books offer good nourishment to the mind, so give the best spiritual or self-development books to the mind to read. Engage it in spiritual discourses so that the body's inactivity decreases and sattva increases. As soon as you find the mind trying to avoid work, immerse it in meaningful and creative work.

This way, tamas can be balanced with the right understanding and awareness. You can further work on your food habits to eliminate lethargy. Avoid consuming food that increases lethargy, like stale, excessively fried and fatty food, fast food, and junk food. Avoid consuming food that is difficult to digest. Stay away from any kind of intoxication. Adopt healthy eating habits and consume wholesome, easily digestible, sattvic, i.e., balanced food. The prospective baby will adopt the same habits as that of the parents. By taking care of these few things, rajas and sattva will increase, and tamas can be balanced.

Q: How can we balance rajas or hyperactivity?

A: People with dominant hyperactive tendencies believe that no work can be done without them. They strongly believe that the world will come to a halt if they do not get up and start working. This conviction is because they consider themselves the doers. Such a self-applauding mindset blinds them. They forget that Mother Nature is the source, channeling ideas and getting Her work done through them. Here, the doer-ship, "I did this, I am doing this… I…, I…, I…" makes them arrogant, restless, and ambitious. To restore and balance this quality, the first thing such people need to do is to stop considering themselves the doer. They need to be liberated from the ego of doer-ship.

They must acknowledge that the Creator is manifesting His work through their body and that the body serves as an instrument in fulfilling His divine plan. Working with this understanding will break their attachment to whatever task they perform. They will neither be attached to its success or failure nor be lured by ambitions. Their mental serenity will remain intact. They will not feel angry, frustrated, or agitated. Apart from this, they also need to practice being in silence for a few moments daily. These moments of stillness will foster detachment and bring poise to their presence. Meditating regularly for a predefined time will help in balancing rajas and keep them detached from the outcome while they work efficiently.

Further, they also need to learn to trust others because people with dominant rajas find trusting others a challenge. For them, delegating work is a daunting task. They fear others might not do the job properly or would not meet the timelines, hence, shoulder it themselves. Women with this attribute cannot share household responsibilities with others. They toil from dawn to dusk, compromising their rest. This habit can be changed by sharing responsibility with everyone. This will ensure the balancing of responsibilities with adequate time for rest and recovery.

Work on balancing rajas and gradually increase sattva. After balancing all the three attributes, you have to further go beyond these three gunas. For this, you need to perform actions without being attached to them and change the intent of self-arrogation behind the efforts, "I am doing this; I will get this benefit and fame." You need to work with a selfless attitude and make it a selfless service.

When you operate with the feeling that the Creator has employed you to do this work, it will benefit the world at large. This will serve as a ladder for the advancement of humanity. If you approach all your tasks with such a selfless attitude and a sense of service, rajas gets balanced, sattva is enhanced, and so is productivity.

In the context of spiritual birthing, this selfless attitude needs to be imbued into the child-bearing endeavor itself. The child that is being birthed is a divine being – a manifestation of God. The parents are selflessly serving the divine purpose of bringing a being of higher consciousness to Earth for the welfare of all.

People with dominant sattva need to remember that they shouldn't be egoistic about their goodness, service, worship, devotion, etc.

Points for reflection

- For life to be happy, healthy, prosperous, peaceful, and creative, it is essential that all the three gunas are balanced. Balance means the three attributes, Rajas, Tamas, and Sattva, are just as much as needed, neither more nor less.
- Observe your 24-hour routine. How much time do you allot to work and entertainment, and how much do you

spend idling? Are you able to render an act of selfless service to others and offer prayers selflessly?
- Fried food, fast food, and junk food increase lethargy. Avoid consuming foods that are difficult to digest; they increase tamas in the body. Hence, working on the quality and quantity of the food you consume is necessary.
- You must raise your awareness whenever the sense of doership arises and remind yourself, "God is getting the work done, using this body as a medium. Its success and failure are dedicated to Him alone; I am only instrumental in carrying out the task." Working with this feeling will break the attachment to karma, leading to liberation from ego, and raise awareness whenever the feeling of doership arises.

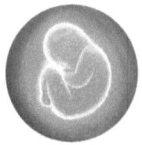

9
See the Truth in Every Situation

Every pregnant woman needs to understand that her unborn baby's brain development is intricately linked to her feelings, thoughts, diet, and environment. Every emotion she experiences, sight, sound, or thought that crosses her mind has a direct impact on the developing baby. Therefore, she needs to be aware.

There are diverse situations in life that surge an array of emotions, giving rise to various mental disorders. Hence, she needs to gain the right understanding to address and eventually dissolve these emotional upheavals. Let us delve deeper into these conditions and explore solutions in the upcoming chapters.

Q: I went out of my way to help some of my relatives. But they just disappeared when I needed their support during my pregnancy; they simply weren't available. They did not even bother to inquire about my well-being. Now, my mind has become hostile towards them. How do I get rid of this negativity?

A: Negativity is an inherent facet of the human mind that recurs often. Generally, people attribute their negativity to others. Have you ever considered the possibility that the other person might be struggling with their own challenges? Assuming that your relative is ignoring you also may not be true; rather, it could be a figment of your imagination.

In such situations, it is important to consider alternative perspectives by posing the following questions to yourself:

1. Is my thinking right, or could it be an illusion, my imaginary story?
2. What are the facts in this situation?
3. What is the truth that differs from the illusion and the facts?

Q: Can you please explain it further?

A: The human mind tends to assume its thoughts and judgments as the absolute truth without any introspection or strong evidence. While such assumptions need not be true, they can also be an illusion. Therefore, before accepting anything as the gospel truth, you should thoroughly introspect whether what you perceive is true or just an illusion. Your mind has convincingly embraced a truth: "I have always helped this person, so they should also help me." So, if they do not help, without knowing the complete truth, the mind will undoubtedly bring doubt.

Q: Then, what is the complete truth?

A: To understand the complete truth, let us first understand the facts in this case. Quite often, surface-level facts can obscure a deeper truth that might not be readily apparent. The fact is that the relatives didn't support you, whatever be the reason. But is it true that they did not really help you?

During pregnancy, you faced some difficulties and anticipated support from your relatives. However, they did not support you. Yet, somehow, you managed to pull yourself through that time. Meanwhile, compelled by circumstances, your husband acquired new skills. He learned to do some household chores, for example, cooking. In the future, as parenthood unfolds, there could be situations where your baby will need your undivided time and attention. So, your husband acquiring new culinary skills would be an added advantage, right? This would ensure a seamless distribution of responsibilities between you and your husband, enhancing your ability to address the needs of an expanding family.

Now, the truth is that even without being supportive, your relatives indirectly helped you in a way no one else could. They helped you build resilience to navigate any adversities of life independently. This also ensured that you need not seek any external assistance and empowered you to adeptly handle life's most difficult situations on your own.

When a father teaches his child to ride a bicycle, he holds the bicycle for a while and then leaves it at the opportune time. This allows the child to ride independently and develop self-reliance. In the same way, nature is also preparing you before entrusting any big responsibility. Nature orchestrates circumstances that enhance your ability and strengthens your capability to shoulder every responsibility that comes your way.

You are now just in the first trimester of your pregnancy. As life unfolds, there could be all kinds of situations. You will have to be self-reliant in dealing with those situations. You cannot raise a child by relying on someone else's aid. So, in this case, the absence of your relatives and their support was nature's most significant help. It empowered you to handle the most difficult crisis skillfully. That's the complete truth.

Sometimes, not receiving help or support is the most significant help. It helps us gain a new and lasting ability to accomplish things independently or seek creative alternatives that foster development.

Points for reflection

- Whenever there is a situation where you find yourself caught in the web of some misunderstanding, assumptions, or negativity towards someone, contemplate using these three questions:
    1) Is my thinking right or could it be an illusion, my imaginary story?
    2) What are the facts in this situation?
    3) Could the truth be something else that I am not comprehending now?
- Nature makes you more capable, strong, and self-reliant through its trials. Therefore, whenever there is any problem or issue, instead of fretting about the probable causes or outcomes, shift your focus to the lessons that you can learn

from the problem. When you face challenges with this understanding, it propels you towards true growth.
- Sometimes, not receiving support is the most significant help. You gain new abilities and become adept at handling the most challenging situations.

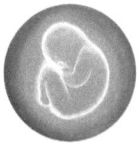

10
Forgiveness to Purify Your Heart

Strange are the ways of the human mind! It forgets and fails to recall things of the recent past or things kept just a while ago, "Oh! Where did I keep my glasses? Where did I keep my mobile?" and so on. Paradoxically, it vividly retains the memories of events from the distant past, re-living them as if they have just transpired. If those incidents were traumatic, they are deeply etched in the human mind. The mind often revisits those painful memories and dives into the abyss of agony that haunts them daily.

The longer a pregnant woman immerses herself in such negative emotions, clings to anger or hateful feelings, and remains in despair or sorrow, the more detrimental it is for the development of the baby. Negative thinking retards the development of the baby's brain in the womb. The happier the mother and the more positive and virtuous life she leads, the better the unborn baby's mental and physical development.

As mentioned in the earlier chapter as well, the baby's state resonates with that of the mother. If the mother is happy, the baby is happy. Similarly, if the mother is sad, the baby gets implanted with seeds of sadness. When the mother is afraid, the feeling of fear is also passed on to the baby. Hence, the mother needs to be careful not to allow or entertain negative thoughts, as they affect the baby's development.

Q: How do we maintain purity and shield the heart from unwanted emotions?

A: There are two aspects to this. The first is to keep the heart pure and the second is to safeguard it from negative emotions. To keep the heart pure, you need to learn to forgive others. A person often holds negative sentiments towards their upbringing, grievances against parents, siblings, etc. "I didn't receive a good upbringing; I didn't enjoy the facilities or get the opportunities I deserved. My sister was jealous of me, etc." Such statements often keep reverberating. These childhood emotions or traumas create lasting impressions and significantly shape an individual's state of mind as they grow. As a result, these unresolved traumas often create discontent. They are neither happy nor satisfied with their present circumstances; hence, they behave accordingly.

You need to acknowledge that parents strive to give their best with the resources available to them. Even if it is not enough for the children, parents usually do all they can. Hence, embrace your childhood and acknowledge the efforts made by your parents by seeking forgiveness and expressing gratitude for the devoted efforts they invested in shaping you into the wonderful human being you are today.

Many factors influence a person's behavioral traits, sculpting their unique persona. It could be their surrounding environment, DNA, family's mindset, their dominant attribute, Rajas, Sattva, Tamas, or their painful memories. Understanding these influences helps recognize the fact that individuals are not solely responsible for their behavior. They are influenced by factors that could be beyond their control. This realization can help you forgive them and contemplate and understand the motives that triggered their behavior.

You need to learn to forgive all those you hold resentment toward and let go of old grudges. You need to safeguard your mind against unwanted polluting thoughts and emotions that add toxicity within and adversely affect the prospective child.

If you let go of your past and move on, most of your problems will automatically resolve. For this, it is imperative to forgive everyone who caused you harm and seek forgiveness from all those whom you would have hurt, knowingly and unknowingly, through your thoughts, feelings, actions, and words.

We all have seen a flowing river. It always remains clean and pure. Conversely, if it stagnates, the water gradually gets polluted and toxic and gets infested with pathogens. This water is not suitable for consumption. Similarly, the mind remains pure as long as thoughts are in motion, i.e., they are flowing. The moment you hold on to unsettling thoughts or emotions, you experience mental stagnation akin to the polluted and toxic water, indicating that the mind is infested.

Therefore, you need to assess the emotions and thoughts with complete awareness, "How could he say this? How dare she do that? I will never forgive them; I will get even with them; I cannot tolerate that person." Such resentful thoughts create mental blocks within, leading to various psychosomatic diseases that can potentially be inherited by the prospective child. It is vital to forgive people to maintain the purity and well-being of your mind, intellect, and emotions. Seek forgiveness for your mistakes and then let go of them. This practice will foster a sense of lightness as if whatever was long held within has finally been cleansed. You will feel stress-free.

Q: How do we seek forgiveness? Is there any method to practice it? What should we do if it is not possible to seek forgiveness from everyone?

A: If you are comfortable seeking forgiveness in person, you should seek forgiveness from them by saying, "If ever I have hurt you, knowingly or unknowingly, with my words, actions, thoughts, or feelings, please forgive me. I will avoid committing such mistakes and will be careful in the future." In this way, you can seek direct apology from your near and dear ones. More importantly, it should be a genuine feeling from the heart, founded on a clear understanding of why seeking forgiveness makes sense.

People are often uncomfortable seeking forgiveness in person and sometimes realize their mistakes much later. In such situations, you can seek forgiveness mentally and forgive them too. By doing this, you will experience remarkable changes in your life. The behavior of those who ignored you or did not behave well with you begins to change. Relations begin to improve, problems are resolved, and everything begins to flow easily in your life. You experience an increased level of inner peace. All this gets transferred to the prospective child as you learn to forgive, thus planting the virtuous seed of forgiveness in the child.

Q: So, can we say that one should seek forgiveness from their parents, siblings, relatives, neighbors, acquaintances, and friends? Should I seek forgiveness from my unborn baby as well?

A: Yes, you should seek forgiveness from all, including your prospective baby. You can seek forgiveness by caressing the womb and saying:

"My dear baby, I seek forgiveness for the impact I've caused by anchoring negative feelings within myself. I promise I will not entertain such negative emotions for anyone in the future. I will give you the required space to develop fully and be happy."

The transformative power of seeking forgiveness cleanses the heart and brings harmony and happiness in relationships; your face will begin to radiate with joy. The warmth and joy radiated by the family members in the harmonious and joyful environment at home enhances the state of happiness in the baby, making it conducive for the baby to unleash its full potential.

Points for reflection

- As the unborn baby's brain development is linked to the emotions of the mother, the child imbibes the same state of mind as the mother. If she remains sad or depressed, exhibiting a tamasic nature, the child will inherit seeds of tamas.

- When a pregnant mother learns to forgive all those for whom she holds resentment and lets go of old grudges, releasing old, accumulated thoughts about incidents by forgiving and seeking forgiveness, she positively influences the prospective child.
- Incredible changes occur once you start forgiving and seeking forgiveness from others. It plants the virtuous seed of forgiveness in the prospective child.

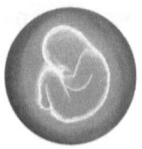

11
Alignment with the Divine Will

The grand blueprint scripted by the Creator determines how a person's life takes shape. Therefore, rejecting one's physical appearance or deformities, amounts to challenging the divine will of the Creator.

The great philosopher Ashtavakra was born with eight physical deformities. According to mythology, when Ashtavakra was in his mother's womb, he pointed out eight errors in his father's rendering of the Vedas. His father got enraged and cursed the unborn baby to be born with eight deformities. Yet, as divine manifestations take remarkable turns, Ashtavakra, despite being born with deformities, attained the zenith of wisdom. King Janaka, of Mithila, who is considered an enlightened master himself, revered Ashtavakra as his Guru.

Q: Some people abandon their unwanted children in orphanages, mainly if the child is born with a deformity or is an unplanned, undesired one. I wonder how these people can do such injustice to their children.

A: This happens when a person wants everything to happen in life as per their personal whims. They have their own subjective criteria of good, bad, right, or wrong for everything. Some people are so obstinate that they accept only those outcomes that align with their personal plans, choices, and desires. If nature offers anything that's contrary to their desires, they dismiss it outright, deeming it inappropriate. In India, unfortunately, such phenomena are more rampant with female children as they are unwanted by their parents and have to face numerous rejections in life because their parents consider them burdensome.

Q: How can one cast away their own child, their own blood?!

A: Yes, one does, because the child is not as they had envisioned or planned for. They fail to acknowledge with the right conscience that the special child is a blessing of the Creator, a divine manifestation of the Creator's intent. They prioritize their own plans and ambitions, blinding themselves to the divine plan of the Creator. You may have heard stories of many great personalities who were abandoned by their parents at birth just because their birth did not conform to their parents' plans and wishes.

Q: Can you share some examples?

A: Sure. You may have heard about Saint Tulsidas, an ardent devotee of Lord Rama and the revered author of the Indian epic Ramcharitmanas. As per the folklore, Saint Tulsidas remained in his mother's womb for twelve months, unlike all other children. He was born a very healthy and strong baby with teeth that were visible at birth. These were all unusual symptoms. Unfortunately, his mother died on the very second day of his birth. His father consulted an astrologer for his horoscope, who deemed him inauspicious after reading the horoscope. First, an abnormal birth, then his mother's demise, and then the astrologer's ominous prediction! The conglomeration of all these resulted in his father abandoning Tulsidas. However, what a saintly child he proved to be. If Saint Tulsidas's father had not abandoned him under the influence of his personal beliefs, he would have felt immense pride in being the father of such a great, pious son.

Similarly, there is a legend about Saint Kabirdas that a weaver couple named Niru and Nima found him floating on a lotus flower in the Lehartara Pond in Kashi, indicating that he was also abandoned after birth. You may have also heard about Karna from the Indian epic Mahabharata and the sacrifice made by his mother, Kunti. Karna suffered a lot due to his mother's fears of social rejection. Yet, he is considered a great philanthropist in history.

Everyone wants their child to be completely healthy, intelligent, and virtuous. But if the child is born with some physical disability, deformity, or mental weakness, do the parents accept the child? Will they be able to give unconditional love to that child? Will they look forward to their child's birth? How happy would they feel? Answers to such questions require deep contemplation and preparation.

Points for reflection

- Most parents generally want everything to happen according to their wishes. If something happens against their will, they curse or blame nature or God and shrug off their responsibility. It is essential to contemplate whether you, too, have done this and introspect that if things are not as per your desires, does that mean that you start behaving differently?
- Contemplate the life of Saint Tulsidas, Saint Kabir, and the great philosopher Ashtavakra. They were abandoned by their parents, and yet they lived by the divine plan that was designed for them by the Creator.

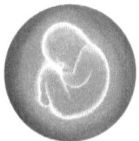

12
Embrace Your Child's Uniqueness

Some questions are such that we do not have the courage to confront them, even in our dreams. People have various apprehensions when it comes to childbirth, which stem from their beliefs.

Mother Nature has a divine plan for all of us, whether we accept it or not. It manifests on its own accord. We can experience true contentment only when we accept and align ourselves with this divine plan. But this cannot be an impromptu action. It requires prior mental and emotional preparation.

Q: What kind of mental and emotional preparation would be required?

A: God has a unique plan for every child; hence, each of them is born differently. They are blessed with a unique body that is destined to accomplish a particular purpose. The child is unique because it aims to work with that body and play a different character in the cosmic drama, just like Sage Ashtavakra.

Prospective parents need to prepare themselves from the very beginning to embrace the Creator's plan for their future children and accept them as divine beings. It is imperative to have a sense of acceptance that every child is a divine incarnation. But due to their apprehensive nature, parents-to-be are unwilling to accept children born differently. They need to understand that there is a unique role assigned to the child, which is going to be a part of their expression.

Disability and weakness exist only in the parents' perceptions and not in the child. Parents need to overcome this weakness in their perception to welcome such divine creations happily. They need to create an environment with ample opportunities for the child to play their unique part and create avenues for their divine expression. In this way, parents will become the best allies in their children's journey to help them fulfil their divine purpose with unconditional support.

Hence, whenever in doubt or sorrow, take inspiration from the great attainments by saints like Jesus, Saint Dnyaneshwar, Saint Tulsidas, Saint Kabir, and Sage Ashtavakra. Keep reminding yourself, "My child is a divine being, who has given me the privilege to be their parent. I promise to enjoy and value their uniqueness and support them wholeheartedly."

Q: I agree with this. Further, I have seen parents who mistreat their children for their weaknesses. They think the children have something amiss, something that is not as per their expectations or so-called "standard" norms. Some parents put so much pressure on their children to earn good grades at school or live up to the family's expectations. This is particularly true with children who are slow learners. Such children go through a lot of frustration and always suffer the feeling of inferiority. What understanding should such parents have?

A: Even if the child is not born according to the parents' wishes, they must passionately accept their offspring. Parents need to offer unwavering and unconditional love and respect to their children. They need to be allies in the child's development, their strong supporter, not their judge or rival. Every parent should develop this mindset before the arrival of the child. It will help promote a healthy start to their formative years.

Saint Soordas, a great devotee of Lord Krishna, was visually impaired from birth, but he possessed a unique gift of narrating the events from Lord Krishna's lifetime as if he had witnessed them first-hand. In today's world, Einstein, one of the icons in physics, was once considered weak mentally. Although his primary education remained incomplete owing to his repeated failures, he went on to become one of the greatest scientists.

Stephen Hawking, one of the topmost scientists, was diagnosed with an early onset of a neuron disease and lost his ability to walk. But with the support from his family, his talent florished. His scientific discoveries changed the world of science forever.

Helen Keller is considered the world's first differently abled graduate. She could not see nor hear, yet not only did she complete her studies, but she proved to be one of America's topmost writers and teachers. This was possible because of the support and cooperation she received from her parents and teachers. Her parents were very proud of her and never felt ashamed of her disabilities.

If there is acceptance for everything one receives from Mother Nature, one's life will be effortless, simple, yet beautiful, and so will the life of one's child(ren). There are many more facets in life where the practice of acceptance is essential. Acceptance is the biggest mantra of a happy life that helps transcend challenges and bring serenity and contentment.

Q: We want to fit everyone into a specific mold. Isn't this the reason for our sorrow?

A: Yes, that's true. The main reason for unhappiness, especially in relationships, is our perceived rejection by the people around us. This world is beautiful owing to its rich diversity, but many people are often unwilling to embrace it fully. Every person is inherently different from the other in their thinking patterns, behavioral traits, qualities, and imperfections, yet they get measured and judged based on the same yardstick. People expect everyone entering their lives to behave according to them. They expect and want people around them to possess the qualities they like and not have those they dislike. They want everything to happen as they wish. If the reality differs from their desires, they get into a sense of rejection. They cannot accept the event as it is; hence, they invite suffering with a baggage of complaints.

For example, they are puzzled over the behaviors of their relatives. "Why is this person acting weird? Why is my child not like others?" They lament even over weather conditions. "I finished my laundry today, but it wasn't sunny enough; why wasn't it sunny? I was about to go out, but it started raining. Why is it Monday? Why couldn't it be a Sunday? Why is there so much traffic? Why is the traffic light red? and so on." The rejection is persistent. This habit of non-acceptance leads to a chronic state of unhappiness throughout their life. This habit is further mirrored by their children as well. They start rejecting things and circumstances. The cycle repeats, and they begin to voice their likes and dislikes. "I want this toy only. I don't want to eat this food. I don't want to wear these clothes," etc. Parents try to guide their children by their preferred methods but often encounter resistance.

Perceived rejection by others invites more sorrow. Parents are disappointed because their children do not follow what they say. Conversely, children feel disheartened when their parents are inattentive to their concerns. The husband complains that the wife does not align with his expectations. The wife expresses her frustration, stating that the husband doesn't care for her. In a professional environment, the manager asserts, "My subordinates don't follow my instructions," whereas the subordinates feel, "My boss is very dominant." They experience discontent as they feel unheard by their superiors.

It is important to understand that nature has made every human being different. They are unique, not only in appearance but also in character. Their thinking, intelligence, and experience all vary from one another. Given these differences, it is important to contemplate if it would be appropriate to expect people to conform to your thoughts. Introspect whether you would be comfortable following someone else's directives and whether you would appreciate if someone else gave instructions or passed judgment on your actions.

Being diverse from each other is what makes us unique. Every human being is complete by themselves, despite variations. No one needs to conform or be like anyone else. Parents need to have this understanding while raising children as well. Each child is and will be, inherently unique and different, and hence they should avoid comparing children.

As emphasized, acceptance is the key. So whatever incidents have happened in your life, whatever has been bestowed by nature, whether in the past or the present, you need to accept the unforgettable memories etched in your mind that are causing distress and let them go. You need to affirm to yourself, "I accept this event, this thing, or this inadequacy or lack in my life." As soon as you accept it, you will observe that the suffering you experience due to them will diminish. Even if it does not vanish completely, it will reduce significantly.

The higher the acceptance towards life, the more stable one feels at the mental level, making them happier and contented, and they can pass on the same feelings to their children.

Points for reflection

- Nature has its divine plan; whether we accept it or not, it works on its own accord. The only way to be happy is to align with nature as soon as possible.
- Every child is a divine creation. Disability and weakness are in people's perception, not in the child. They are blessed with a unique body and are destined to accomplish the Creator's unique purpose. Hence, parents need to work on their own resistance and welcome the divine creation happily.
- Nature has made every human being unique, and they are complete by themselves, even though there are variations in their appearances and behavior. Parents need to embrace this understanding while interacting with their children. Regardless of the child's traits, they are inherently unique, and there's no need to compare or judge.
- The more the acceptance towards life increases, the more stable one feels at the mental level, making them happier and contented, and they then pass on the same feelings to their children.

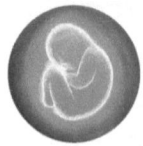

13
The Feeling of Abundance

Women who live in the feeling of abundance during their prenatal period remain happy and contented. They have full faith that Mother Nature will take care of them and their prospective baby. The same trust and sentiment also get ingrained in the baby in the womb, instilling a feeling of abundance right from the formative months. Every prospective mother should impart such values to her unborn baby in the womb itself.

Q: The feeling of fulfillment arises only when we have enough. But we don't always get enough of what we need in life. I always feel a sense of lack, sometimes of money or resources, sometimes of good clothes, or good relations or trustworthy friends. I believe the feeling of contentment is elusive as no one in the world has everything; no one seems happy.

A: When it rains, it rains all over the city, but does everyone get drenched in that rain? No! Not all get wet. Some are spared from getting wet because they have an umbrella or find shelter.

If people who did not get wet said, "There wasn't enough rain, we didn't get wet," then would you blame the rain? Is it the rain's fault? The clouds showered the same water on everyone without bias, but only those who did not take shelter under an umbrella received rain.

Q: Agreed, but so many people struggle with the feeling of lack and poverty. Then how can we feel abundant? And what does taking shelter under an umbrella mean?

A: It is just a matter of perspective and belief one holds. Mother Nature abundantly provides for all. There is more than enough of everything for everyone. This is one of the laws of nature, known as the Law of Abundance. But people do not believe in this law. They are under the influence of their wrong beliefs that there isn't enough. For example, they hold strong beliefs such as, "I am always short of money; even if I do receive money, it barely stays with me." This is a limiting belief that acts as an umbrella, blocking the shower of blessings and abundance.

If one persistently feels strapped financially, no matter how much money they have, it will always seem insufficient. Even a minimal expenditure will trigger a negative perception of loss, "My money is gone." Such people fail to recognize the fact that they have received something in exchange for that money, like goods, groceries, education, health, and so on. Such people even treat children's school fees and money spent on household groceries as an expense. On the contrary, people with an abundance mindset consider it an investment because they know this money will bring good health and education to their families.

The same applies to relationships as well. Many people feel unloved and unacknowledged by their family. If they persistently shield themselves with the umbrella of such negative thoughts, then how will anyone's love and respect reach them? Their complaint is, "Nowadays, the world lacks good, trustworthy people." They need to understand that holding on to the umbrella of such a negative mindset will prevent good people from entering their lives. On the contrary, when they start believing in the Law of Abundance and change their mindset with the right understanding, the umbrella dissolves, allowing blessings to flow in their lives.

Mother Nature is always ready to provide everything; all one needs is unwavering faith in it. When you imbue feelings of harmony, love, health, peace, and prosperity into relationships, everything else is bound to flow. You need to cultivate a sense of abundance in all aspects. You can keep affirming to yourself, "There is more than enough. All my desires are already manifesting in my life," and leave the rest to the benevolence of nature.

Here is a short story that will help you to understand this concept. There was a happily married woman who desired to conceive but encountered challenges in doing so. She underwent various medical treatments but to no avail. The doctors were perplexed because even though she was medically fit to conceive, they could not diagnose any cause for her infertility. What was amiss then?

The limiting factor was her wrong thoughts.

What an irony; our medical science can only detect the deficiency in the body, not the deficiency in thoughts and feelings.

The woman had created a mental barrier within herself through wrong thoughts, blocking the manifestation of her earnest desire. You may wonder how. Whenever she thought about her prospective child, her thoughts echoed, "I don't know whether we will be able to take care of our child. We lack the necessary facilities. Our expenses will increase, and the budget will go haywire. Our income is not sufficient to raise a child. What will happen if there is a significant increase in the medical expenses? How will we arrange the funds to send our child to a good school? Education is expensive these days," and so forth.

Thus, she did not perceive the prospective child as a gift from God but unconsciously considered it an impending cause of expenses. As the days passed, her apprehensions and negative notions about the child's future and associated expenses just grew. She was unaware that her thoughts were steering her away from the feeling of abundance. Her own thoughts were blocking the arrival of her prospective child. If she were told, "You are blocking your child from entering your life," she would not agree because this is a force that works in the invisible realm.

This is the Law of Nature. It states that if you live in the feeling of abundance for the things you desire and are open to possibilities, they will surely manifest in your life.

Your vibrations change when you change your feelings, making you receptive, and everything becomes easily available.

Points for reflection

- The feeling of abundance is a value that every mother should ingrain within her child in the womb and open the path to happiness.
- Have faith that everything is abundant for you and the prospective child – love, health, peace, money, harmonious relationships – everything.
- If the feeling of abundance seems elusive, you need to check your thoughts. You must shift your thoughts and feelings towards abundance by affirming that there is more than enough for everyone and embed this feeling in the unborn baby.

PART II

Instilling Higher Values in the Baby

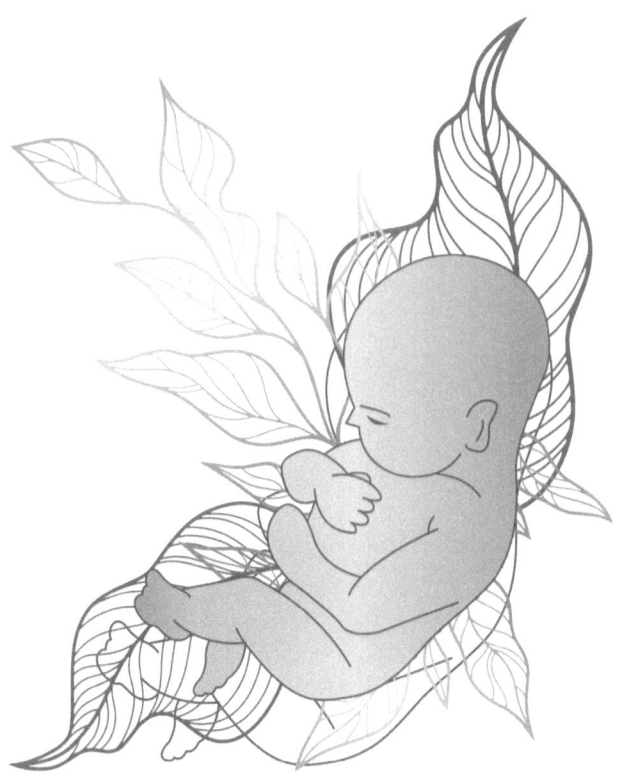

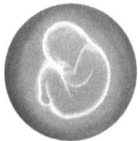

14

Center Your Focus to Instill Virtues

The human mind is made up of two parts: the Outer Mind and the Inner Mind. All our conscious thoughts, perceptions, and awareness of our surroundings occur in the outer mind, also known as the conscious mind. The inner mind functions behind the scenes, influencing our thoughts, feelings, and behavior through stored memories, beliefs, and instincts. It is also referred to as the subconscious mind. The outer mind typically comprises around 10% of our mind, while the subconscious mind makes up 90%.

Q: I am curious to know how the subconscious mind works.

A: The conscious mind, as the name suggests, functions while we are awake and conscious. But the subconscious mind operates even when we are in deep sleep. This mind is closer to the Universal or Collective Mind. Whatever we strongly believe in function as seeds in the fertile soil of our inner mind, and we see the outcomes of those beliefs in our lives. Everything we feed into our subconscious mind starts materializing in the physical realm.

If, for some reason, a person firmly believes that they do not get support from people or life is a never-ending struggle, then the power of their subconscious mind turns this belief into reality. Indeed, they will experience non-cooperation and struggles in life. On the contrary, if they hold the belief that everything in their life comes easily and smoothly, they will experience that their lives are shaped accordingly. This is the power of the subconscious mind, a genie that will convert whatever you have faith on into reality.

The mother's subconscious mind is deeply connected to the baby's. Every strong positive or negative thought that the mother's subconscious mind holds on to or believes, leaves a lasting impression on the baby's subconscious mind. It gets ingrained in the form of a sanskar. The baby's subconscious mind absorbs every emotion the mother experiences, which then shapes its life. Hence, it is imperative to instill the right values during pregnancy.

Q: How do you train this powerful subconscious mind?

A: Every mother has this golden opportunity to ingrain the best qualities in her child. To be able to do so, she needs to alter her thought patterns, emotions, and perspectives first. The qualities she focuses on, leave a lasting impression on the child's subconscious. When she focuses not on others' blemishes but on their virtues, not on scarcity but on abundance, the same gets etched on the baby's subconscious mind. These then manifest in the child's life later.

Every mother aspires that her children embody higher values and virtues, but for this to happen, she must focus on internalizing these qualities and values herself.

Q: I tend to recall all my positive experiences when exposed to good content. But when I attend social gatherings or visit my hometown, I meet and interact with many relatives. Some are always scrutinizing my flaws or are on the lookout for my failures. They are always eyeing an opportunity to taunt me despite being a bundle of imperfections themselves. This spoils my mood, creating a negative impact on the baby as well. How do I maintain positivity in such situations?

A: A mother-to-be should consider the prenatal period an opportunity to gather and internalize virtuous qualities in her routine for her prospective child. It is entirely her choice to either focus on the virtues or the flaws of others. Consciously or unconsciously, the feelings she harbors towards her family members, relatives, or people around her get impregnated in her unborn baby, who absorbs these feelings in their subconscious mind, that reflect in their behavior later.

There's another perspective to this. There is not a single person in the world devoid of good qualities, perhaps less, but they undoubtedly possess at least one good quality. The key is to identify and focus on those or that one good quality, even in those you dislike or perceive as negative. Consider the quality you focus on as if you are invoking and inviting it in your child. So, if you are centering your attention on the negatives of those people, you are inviting those negativities for your future child. Hence, as a mother, you must focus on goodness in everyone you meet and deliberately overlook their flaws. Doing so will craft positive impressions on the baby's future.

Imagine the child's subconscious mind as a shopping basket wherein you have to place good qualities selectively. All these qualities can be easily found in the people around you; you only need to focus on identifying them, and the rest will naturally unfold. The mother is the link between her family members, relatives, and her child. She can cultivate feelings of love, self-esteem, and mutual respect for all relatives in the child.

Here's an assignment you can do. Contemplate your closest relatives and favorite people individually and identify five virtues in each of them. Write down those virtues and repeatedly center your focus on them. Even if you can practice this with ten people, you have amassed fifty qualities for your child.

Q: Yes, I agree with this. There are so many people who are a goldmine of qualities. I greatly respect them and want my child to possess those qualities. But I may not be able to meet all of them. Is there a solution to this?

A: It is not necessary for the person to be in front of you to focus on their qualities. You can contemplate and meditate on their qualities. In the Indian tradition, you pin up posters and photographs of inspiring personalities in the expectant mother's room so that she can focus on their qualities. These qualities are then awakened in the children as well. Not only pregnant women but even children, teenagers, and adults put up pictures of their role models in their rooms or keep them in their wallets and read their autobiographies.

You will often find pictures of Lord Krishna in His infant state in the homes of an expectant mother in India. The reason is to awaken His qualities in the mother and her prospective child. This is also the science behind idol worship: to invoke the divine attributes of the deities in the subconscious mind so that they manifest in your life.

You can develop an action plan to adopt and awaken the best qualities in your child. For this, you will have to sit with your family and decide which qualities you all would want in your prospective baby. Once done, you can put up pictures of inspiring souls depicting those qualities, such as the Buddha for Peace, Lord Rama for his moral decorum, Mother Teresa for her compassion and so on. In this way, you can create a vision board and hang it in your house where it is visible to all. You can plant these seeds in the child by repeatedly contemplating these qualities.

Points for reflection

- The qualities or shortcomings an expectant mother focuses on are passed on to her baby through her subconscious mind. Hence, she should always focus on virtues during pregnancy.
- The feelings the expecting mother harbors for her family members are absorbed by her unborn baby. Hence, cultivating love, honor, and respect for all is important.
- List at least five qualities of each of your close relatives and contemplate them. Doing so will emboss these qualities in the child's subconscious mind and manifest in their life.
- Create a vision board with pictures depicting all the qualities you expect in the child and observe them repeatedly.

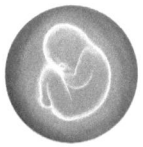

15
Conscious Conversation with the Baby

In ancient times, sages, who led family life, often described the bond between the mother and the baby growing in her womb as akin to two peas nestled in a pod. They share one stomach, and their eyes and ears are also interconnected, signifying the unity of their senses, mind, and intellect.

As we have been reading, the baby is nourished with what the mother eats. It listens to what the mother listens to. What the mother feels, creates lasting impressions in the baby's formative mind. Whatever the mother speaks, the prospective baby perceives as the final verdict, eventually shaping their thoughts.

Hence, consciously engaging in healthy and positive conversation with the baby through these senses and sharing meaningful and good information and higher values is important. This is the primary means of instilling prenatal values. The family should be mindful that the baby is absorbing everything being said directly to the baby or about the baby. It may not sound logical as it all happens in the invisible realm.

Q: Is it really possible that the baby in the womb can hear what we say or listen to our conversations? We need a body, and more so, we need mature ears to listen to anyone. If someone is in another room, they cannot hear what we say; how can the baby hear when it is inside the womb?

A: There's a well-known tale from the Indian epic Mahabharata. It states that once Prince Arjuna was explaining one of the important warfare techniques, the Chakravyuh battle formation, to his then-pregnant wife Subhadra. Chakravyuh means a maze, and Prince Arjuna was explaining the strategies to enter and traverse through the Chakravyuh. The baby in her womb, Abhimanyu, was also listening to this conversation. However, while she was listening, Subhadra drifted into sleep amid the conversation and stopped listening. As a result, Abhimanyu missed out on the strategies needed to come out of the maze.

Q: Yes, I have heard this story. I felt it was a fictional part of the story. How can a child who is yet to come into this world, who does not understand language, who does not yet have a fully developed ear, listen to everyone?

A: Every word carries energy and feelings. Regardless of the understanding of the language, the feelings and energy of the words get relayed from one being to another. The baby's body may still be developing, yet it is a complete being, just like all of us. The child may not know the language, but it can capture the essence of whatever is perceived through the mother's senses. The baby comprehends and stores all the feelings of everything felt and spoken in its memories.

Q: How can we talk to the baby in the womb?

A: You can talk to the baby just as you talk to anyone else directly, i.e., in person or over the phone. You can imagine this as if you are calling the baby on the phone and start talking. You don't have to doubt whether it is listening or not, whether it is responding or not. You need to have this conviction that the baby is listening and responding to every word you say.

Q: What can we talk to the baby in the womb?

A: You can talk about almost everything with the baby in the womb, which you would otherwise speak to a child. You can ask how it is doing. You can share how your day was. How happy or excited you are for its presence in your life, how eager you are to see it, how special the baby is to you. You can express everything that you feel for the baby. You can also share a memorable incident of your life, your childhood memories, dreams, plans, and ambitions. Share everything with the firm belief that it is listening to you as if it were your soulmate, who is close to you, standing before you. Have faith in the connection and communicate with the conviction that your words and emotions resonate with the little bundle of joy growing inside you.

You can also narrate inspiring stories or read biographies of magnanimous people. You can give positive affirmations, happy and healthy vibes to the baby. You can share words of wisdom, recite divine couplets, hymns, bhajans, etc., and sow the seeds of spiritual awakening within the baby.

Q: Please help me by providing some examples of good vibes that can be given to the baby.

A: Sure. There are no fixed rules to it, but to practice this, you can lovingly place your hand on your womb and feel the baby's touch. The father can participate, too. By doing this, the baby will feel the touch of the mother and father together. This will create a beautiful bond between the three. This is how you can give good vibes or beliefs to the baby and then say:

> "My dear child,
> I/ We wish to tell you how much I/we love you. I/we care a lot for you. I am delighted that you are here. I am with you every moment, feeling and caring for you. You are completely safe in my womb. You are developing well, and we will continue to give our best, which is essential for your right development. May you always be joyous and peaceful."

Such positive talk will give the baby a feeling of warmth, faith, and security. Similarly, you can converse with the baby to awaken divine qualities.

> "My dear child,
> We are so grateful to have you in our lives! You are a divine gift God has bestowed on us. You are an integral part of the

Creator, a divine creation. You possess divine qualities and are incarnating here to express them. You are being born to accomplish the extraordinary work of God. Your life will be divinely guided, and you are fully capable of receiving that guidance.

Your heart is brimming with love and compassion for all. You are always ready to help and serve others. Your wisdom and consciousness are awakened, which will empower you to make the right decisions in life. You respect everyone and, in turn, garner respect from all. You find joy in the happiness of others. Hence, people around you feel happy in your joyous presence. You are a unique confluence of knowledge and devotion, adorned with divine qualities like humility, compassion, courage, and determination. Your arrival on earth will benefit this world and society in many ways, and we are immensely proud of you. May you always remain peaceful and joyous, my dear child."

Q: Wow! This is an excellent way of communicating. But can we really develop so many qualities just by speaking to the baby in the womb?

A: Yes, of course. The child will develop according to the beliefs given to it. And through the right communication, healthy beliefs can be ingrained in the baby right from conception.

Points for reflection

- The baby in the womb can hear us. Hence, consciously engage in healthy and meaningful conversation with it.
- One can talk to the baby in the womb the same way as they would with any other human being.
- One can convey a sense of security, virtues, wisdom, and positive beliefs to the baby through positive conversations with the baby.

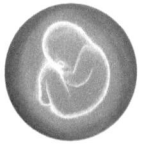

16
Impact of Gender Discrimination

In India, some people believe that the preservation and continuance of the family legacy and its prestige solely depends on the birth of a son. The son is envisioned as the sole member who can or will lend support, comfort, and solace to parents as they age. Hence, to materialize this aspiration, to-be parents meticulously follow some customary practices like chanting mantras, performing certain rituals, offering prayers, and vowing charity.

Q: To what extent is this prejudice for the male child justified? After all, what is destined to happen will manifest. Once conceived, how can that be changed?

A: The manifestation of gender is entirely a natural process based on science that happens at the time of conception. It cannot change. Now, imagine if the baby in the womb is a girl and hears these mantras and prayers being chanted by parents aspiring a male child. What will her emotional state be when she realizes her parents' desire? While she is absorbing her parents' emotions, it might make her feel unwanted and give her a sense of rejection. She will experience intense turbulence within, sensing that her identity as a girl is unacceptable to her parents. These sentiments of rejection will be the cause of deep sorrow for that innocent, tender baby while still in the womb.

All aspiring parents need to understand that refuting a baby for its gender leaves an enduring scar on the baby's psyche. They experience a deep sense of rejection and profound sadness. This emotional turmoil can lead to accumulating distortions, developing an inferiority complex, and deep resentment within the unborn baby.

Chanting mantras and offering prayers during the prenatal period is good, but the key is to practice it mindfully. The purpose of prayers, chanting mantras, or reading spiritual literature should not be gender-centric or to predict the baby's gender. Rather, practice them to convey benevolence, nurture the baby's well-being, and envelop the child in love and care, irrespective of the gender.

You should thank the baby for gracing you with the privilege of parenthood. This bundle of joy is the source of your happiness. Its arrival will bring a wealth of learnings and experiences, enhance and deepen your understanding of life, and develop new qualities within you. You can share your feelings with the unborn baby in simple words. Here's how:

> "My dear child,
> Thank you so much for gracing our lives with your presence. Whoever you are, you are perfect in every way; you are the best.
> You embody purity; you are akin to the Buddha; you are a holy, sacred, and divine creation. You are one with the Creator. Your arrival is a sacred contribution to elevate the consciousness of the Earth.
> We wholeheartedly welcome and accept you for who and how you are. We love and respect you. May your journey be joyous and happy eternally."

Q: Expectant mothers often receive blessings from their relatives for giving birth to a male child in Asian countries. They also suggest certain practices and rituals believed to ensure the birth of a boy. This stirs irritation and resentment towards such people. What can we do in such situations?

A: You need not hold any resentment or hatred towards anyone. Such thinking often stems from their personal experience and surroundings. Their environment has been the biggest catalyst in shaping their perceptions about a girl child. However, we need to acknowledge that with time, there has been a positive shift in the attitude and perspective of the new generation, and these beliefs are now becoming redundant.

The best would be to divert your focus from the negativity. Think of all those relatives who trigger these negative emotions by bringing them into your field of attention. Now, consciously identify five positive qualities in them and focus on those qualities. As mentioned in the preceding chapter, you can gather flowers of virtues from each one to weave a garland of virtues for your prospective child. Accept everyone as they are and prioritize self-care because this is your responsibility towards your child(ren).

Points for reflection

- Parents must refrain from gender-based discrimination. It can impede the mental and physical growth of unborn baby.
- If the baby faces rejection based on its gender or for any other reason, it negatively impacts the baby's psyche, causing emotional distress.
- One should divert their focus from negativity and prioritize self-care as this is your responsibility towards your child(ren).

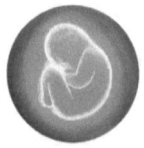

17

Appreciation and Gratitude

Can you imagine a divine child?

Picture a gentle, innocent, smiling child – a soul that emanates love and goodwill for all. A soul that bears no enmity or ill-will towards anyone, but radiates only love, joy, peace, and goodwill for the betterment of society.

These attributes form the essence of a divine child. Pregnancy is an opportunity to ingrain the seeds of these values, laying the foundation for a divine manifestation. This does not necessitate significant effort but indeed demands a shift in one's understanding and vision.

Q: People do not want to give birth to divine children. Most people hold beliefs such as it's too idealistic a notion or that the world is not ready for virtuous people as only the shrewd and opportunists can survive. These beliefs make them fear that an innocent child is vulnerable to exploitation and may never be successful in the world. There's also a fear that such a child may renounce worldly pursuits and become a hermit. These thoughts can make parents uncertain about giving birth to a child with divine qualities, who may choose the unconventional path in life.

A: This voice echoes the insecurities hidden within a mother. Much as the mother may revere virtuous saints, she worries that if her child becomes one, the child will ultimately leave her. She fears detachment. With this, she also imagines a scenario where her child, with the acquired wisdom and maturity, will begin to analyze and challenge societal norms like dowry, bribery, corruption, and religious hypocrisy. She anticipates that her child may even rebel against the family. This dilemma highlights the challenge of imbibing higher values that parents may not fully understand, and their own fears and misgivings over various issues.

For example, Prince Siddhartha's life took a twist owing to his father's insecurities. His father, King Shuddhodhana, tried to keep Siddhartha away from the unavoidable truths of life. But as you may know, this resulted in the Prince relinquishing his royal comforts and embracing the life of a recluse in pursuit of the ultimate wisdom. Had Siddhartha received a righteous and balanced upbringing, he could have become a Rajarishi – an enlightened being and also an effective king, like the revered King Janaka. Parents are the architects of their children's lives. They will have to extensively enhance their understanding and work on any such anxieties or skewed perceptions ideally before conception so that they do not hinder their child's divine expression.

Q: What is the understanding we must adopt to create an environment conducive to nurture a divine or virtuous child?

A: First we must develop a deep sense of appreciation for everything around us. This quality is inherent in children from the moment they are born. Observe a baby exploring its surroundings and notice the marvel in its eyes. Observe how it is fascinated by the beautiful dew drops on the leaves. Babies are in awe, looking at the wonders of nature. Watching their pure, innocent smile and the sheer joy when they touch and experience the marvels of nature is mesmerizing. The curiosity in their eyes, watching those tiny insects and ants, their fascination while watching the beautiful birds, butterflies, and the captivating beauty of the flowers, is an example of their unfiltered natural appreciation for the existence of the beauty of the nature around them.

Man is lost to this beauty that unfolds each day, every moment. The graceful blossoming of flowers, the ascent of the majestic sun, the cosmic ballet of the moon and stars, everything unfolds so beautifully, yet most of us are indifferent to all this. We chase material acquisitions, take things for granted, and create a void in our lives. Since we fail to appreciate the daily miracles, we feel discontented and yearn for more material happiness.

Living with such adults, children, who innately appreciate nature, drift away from their inherent inclination of observing the wonders of nature. Their true experience of life begins to fade as they, too, start struggling to cope with life's pressures and expectations.

It's time to shift perspectives. By observing the Creator's divine creations, you can honor the minutest wonders. You will feel the divine presence everywhere, in every little thing. This experience invites you to recognize, appreciate, and acknowledge the artistry of the ultimate craftsman and the divinity that flows into every creation. It fills you with immense gratitude and inspires divine creativity. You may even write beautiful poems, hymns, and other forms of thanksgiving in praise of all creation.

Appreciation increases your receptivity to divine grace, resulting in increased positivity. This new approach gives a unique perspective to your child. Hence, from now on, start appreciating the good you see around you, in nature and people.

Q: Wow! Thank you for throwing light on what we miss seeing. Is there anything else we need to bear in mind to manifest a divine child?

A: Only half the work is done with appreciation. In addition to this, you need to learn to express gratitude for everything that deserves gratitude.

Gratitude to that child who chose you as its mother, gratitude to this body that cared for you and the prospective child. Gratitude to nature for all the elements like air, water, fire, earth, and space that contribute to your existence. Gratitude to all whose presence keeps your and everyone's life on track and running smoothly. Gratitude for all the qualities, skills, prosperity, and health you possess and for all you desire and receive. Gratitude also for those desires you didn't wish for and yet manifested by grace. Express gratitude to the Creator and Mother Nature for every blessing in life.

Q. What is the best way to practice gratitude?

A. You may practice Gratitude Meditation. There is no fixed method for this. It can be practiced with open eyes even while walking or sitting quietly in one place.

Glance at your surroundings and see the blessings showered on you – this life as a human being, your physical body, good health, career, harmonious relationships, friends, home, comforts, spiritual associations, the grace of being blessed with a Spiritual Guide or Guru, and most importantly, the divine bundle of joy growing within you.

You can also list everything you have been graced with – a beautiful home, parents, family, good neighbors and co-workers, resources, water, food, education, security, good facilities, help, etc. Express your heartfelt gratitude to the Creator for every grace.

Next is manifesting your desires with the power of gratitude. You can visualize the desires you wish to manifest. Visualize the pleasant changes they will bring to your life and be in that feeling for a few moments. Imagine you are being graced with that desire and anchor that feeling within. Thank the Creator and express your heartfelt gratitude in anticipation of that special grace. This practice will increase your receptivity to receiving these blessings, which will then manifest sooner.

As you cultivate this habit of expressing gratitude, a cascade of unnoticed blessings will unravel. The realization that the Creator has abundantly provided everything, yet you never acknowledged, will dawn. This meditation will uplift you from all the disappointments of life and perceived scarcities. The key is to start expressing gratitude whenever you see or feel a sense of lack in life. You will witness an immediate transformation in your feelings and feel an inherent abundance within. This feeling of gratitude will act as a magnetic force to attract more blessings into your life.

Practice such meditations with the awareness that even the unborn baby in your womb is participating with you. While you observe and appreciate something, envision the baby's perspective integrating with yours. Feel that the baby is also appreciating the world alongside you through its own yet unseen gaze. When you experience a blessing and feel grateful, the baby also shares gratitude with you in its own way. When you thank the Creator, the baby and you also connect in divine harmony.

Points for reflection

- Pregnancy is an opportunity for divine manifestation. Parents need to work on their own insecurities, develop their understanding, and let go of fears about a divine child.
- Parents need to teach their child(ren) the values of appreciation and gratitude.
- Parents need to ingrain the habit of acknowledging and appreciating everything in the world where the baby is arriving. For this, the parents will have to start appreciating things themselves.
- Parents can cultivate this habit of acknowledging and expressing gratitude by bringing all blessings into their sphere of attention and thanking the Creator.
- While practicing gratitude, the mother must envision her baby acknowledging, appreciating, and expressing gratitude alongside her.

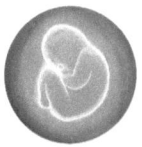

18
Sow the Seeds of Benevolence

Benevolence and compassion are indispensable divine qualities that everyone should possess because only then can one fulfill their duty as a human being. These qualities aren't just nice to have; they're essential to our very nature. By embracing them, we keep our minds free from negativity and ensure the purity of our intentions towards others.

Q: In one of the discourses, I heard that the very act of gazing at someone can become a prayer, a meditation, transforming us and the other person. Can I get more clarity on this?

A: Yes, of course, such a benevolent gaze is possible. We all have two eyes. So let us say our one eye can be a conduit of love and the other an envoy of compassion. With this understanding, consider looking at someone as not merely an act of seeing; instead, showering them with bright rays of love and compassion. This shift in understanding will elevate one's vision into a state of prayer and blessing.

The wise gaze of great saints and spiritual masters is always infused with love and benevolence. This is why people yearn for a glimpse of them, believing their gaze has the transformative power to heal and uplift them. This happens because their consciousness and healing or uplifting sentiments reach others through their gaze, deeply touching the very fiber of their being.

Hence, changing the perspective with which you look at others and infusing your gaze with love and compassion is imperative. To cultivate this habit, you can include the following steps whenever you look at someone.

Suppose you are going to the office or are walking on the streets, in the market, or at home; infuse your gaze with compassion, good wishes, love, and kindness. Keep an intention that your gaze is a catalyst that will transform the people around you, making them healthy, elevating their consciousness, and gracing them with blessings.

If there are any negative feelings like anger or hatred towards someone, bring them into your sphere of awareness. Now, picture them sheathed in bright rays of kindness and compassion in your mind's eye. Imagine radiating positive intentions, heartfelt blessings, and goodwill in their direction. Now, continue to visualize them in your mental space and affirm, "You are noble. You are humble. You are capable. You are wise. You are healthy. You are a seeker of truth. You are a symbol of purity. You embody perfection. You radiate these virtues, and all the negativities of the mind are being dispelled." In this way, you can send uplifting wishes to all.

You not only impregnate your gaze for others but also for yourself and the baby. Bring yourself and the baby into your sphere of awareness. Imagine yourself and the baby immersed in an aura of bright healing light and visualize love, kindness, and compassion being showered on both of you. Repeat these affirmations to yourself and the baby, "You are pure. You are wise like the Buddha. You are humble. You embody perfection. You are imbued with vibrant health. You are the master of divine qualities." This is called a healing gaze.

In this way, altering your gaze with this newfound perspective benefits at least three people—first is you, second, the baby, and third, the other person. You will observe positive changes in the other person.

Q: What should we do when we encounter people for whom envisioning benevolence becomes challenging?

A: You must practice the same thing with those people, too.

Q: But if someone constantly engages in wrongdoings, cheats, and causes distress, how can we see them with love and compassion? Sometimes, office colleagues cause distress, or the house help routinely skips work, is late, or does shoddy work. In such situations, it seems impossible.

A: Always remember one thing: there's no one in the world who doesn't deserve the gaze of benevolence and compassion. If someone behaves in a particular manner, it simply means they are unwell, maybe not physically, but they may be mentally or emotionally unwell. They need to receive even more compassion to be healed. Hence, you need to do what is right with such people. Consider it an act of service.

For example, if employees, subordinates, or colleagues keep making excuses or avoiding work, they will face the consequences someday. You may need to make tough decisions or take strong actions, but they need not be out of anger or hatred. Regardless of the external conditions, you need to maintain the feeling of compassion within. Nurture love and compassion, especially for all those you perceive as negative or unfavorable, those you dislike, or those with flaws. Now, individually bring all of them into your sphere of awareness and visualize enveloping them in the bright radiance of love and compassion. Develop the habit of showering rays of love and compassion to the extent your gaze goes and to whoever you see. You must encompass good wishes and happy thoughts in your gaze for all. When your heart and vision are filled with blessings, your gaze transcends into prayer and meditation.

As for the house help, you can warn them and prompt them to admit or confess their mistakes. If necessary, you may even need to lay them off work. However, you should be clear from within that they are under the invisible influence of a negative mind and therefore deserve a gaze of love and kindness. Even while you reprimand them, maintain benevolent feelings toward them. You must take the necessary actions as it is your rightful duty, but continue to shower positive rays and affirm, "You are pure. You are a child of God. May you always receive blessings. May you develop divine qualities within you."

With consistent practice, you will notice that, with time, you do not get annoyed or angry with anyone. Your reactions have changed, and the resentment and frustrations of the mind have reduced. You are becoming pure, wiser, and righteous within; your baby, too, will be born with these qualities.

Now that you have understood the importance of seeing everyone through the lens of love and compassion, you should practice this meditation for some time daily. Turn by turn, bring all the people you know, the baby and yourself, into your sphere of awareness and visualize bright rays of love and compassion falling on them. All the bitterness in your mind will wash away, making you feel lighter and better.

After this, the next step is to amplify your prayer to the highest level towards completion.

Q: What does amplifying prayer mean? Isn't just praying enough?

A: Amplifying prayer would mean enhancing the power of prayer and giving completion to them. A small addition to your prayer will elevate the power of your prayer manifold. Whenever you pray for yourself and the baby, all you have to do is include everyone else in your prayer and seek blessings for all. By doing so, the impact of your prayers will be amplified, reaching its highest level and attaining completion.

For example, you pray – "O God! May my child receive good health."

You might as well pray – "O God! May my child and all children receive good health."

Suppose you pray, "O God! May I receive respect, dignity, and prosperity."

Instead, pray, "O God! May everyone, including me, receive respect, dignity, and prosperity."

Suppose you pray, "O God! Let the light of truth and wisdom shine in my life."

Instead, pray, "O God! Let the light of truth and wisdom shine in everyone's life, including me."

In this way, you include everyone in your prayers. "May we all receive blessings and gain wisdom, devotion, good health, divine virtues, abundance, and prosperity." With this practice, your prayer will transform into one for the well-being of all. It will become a selfless prayer. These values of wishing for the well-being of all will be imbibed in the baby right from the formative years, with wondrous results in its earthly life. The baby's life will be evocative and a catalyst in bringing love, peace, and harmony to the world.

Points for reflection

- The child needs to imbibe the quality of seeing every living being in this world through the lens of love and compassion right from the beginning so that they become a good human being.
- For this, the parents will have to change their perspective. Whoever they see, they must look at them through the lens of love and compassion. In this way, their gaze will become a prayer, a meditation.
- Parents need to visualize themselves and their baby with this new healing vision.
- If you dislike someone or get angry, you need to bring them into your sphere of awareness and envelop them in rays of love and compassion.
- Include everyone in your prayer and amplify the power of your prayer, making it selfless and universal. This practice will bring wondrous results, making the baby a catalyst for love, peace, and harmony.

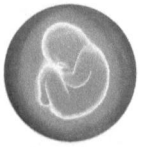

19

Free the Child from Your Pain

It is often observed that parents harbor bitterness within, which they usually manifest as anger towards their children. They blame everyone around them, and the whole world appears deceitful to them. The world appears to them according to the beliefs they hold on to. If they have no faith in goodness, they can remain perpetually immersed in pain and suffering.

Q: A couple in my neighborhood has a skeptical view of Garbh Sanskar. They say, "If a pigeon sits with closed eyes in front of a cat, it does not mean the cat doesn't exist, and the pigeon is not in danger!" In other words, they suggest that Garbha Sanskar amounts to closing one's eyes in the face of potential dangers. These talks of love, positivity, and compassion are all baseless. Nowadays, even our relatives do not offer support, expecting support from others is even more farfetched. Sometimes, children also leave their parents when they grow up. No matter how many virtues are imbued in the child, they will learn from what they see in this world and follow the prevalent societal norms." I am confused after hearing all this. Please shed some light on this.

A: Let us try to understand this through an analogy of a pen and a pencil. One day, pen and pencil met in a library. They started talking to each other and felt they had so much in common. They had "pen" in common, not just in their names, but also figuratively since they had "pain" in common. Both decided to get married based on this commonality. Doesn't it often happen that two individuals cross paths sharing similar habits, likes, and dislikes, and believe they are an ideal match for each other and contemplate marriage?

Pen-Pencil shared the same sentiments and decided to get married. After their wedding, they both collectively created a Pen (read, Pain) drive. A Pen drive is a device that stores information or data like important text files, videos, audios, photos, etc. So, they created a common drive and populated it with their common pains and struggles. They had the potential to formulate a cure for their common afflictions that would have emptied the pain drive. But instead, they chose differently.

Further, the painful data in this pen (pain) drive was transferred to their child because, during pregnancy, they watched, read, and listened to all that was stored in the same pen (pain) drive. Had Pen and Pencil formulated the cure for their afflictions and worked on resolving them, resulting in emptying the data in the drive, the child would have been free from inheriting their pain. Pen and Pencil inadvertently burdened their child with pain, something that could have been avoided.

Q: Could you please explain this analogy in more detail?

A: When two people unite in marriage, they bring along their distinct set of beliefs and thinking patterns. They possess their own perspectives about life and the world, both positive and negative.

Now, imagine the scenario when two individuals with negative mindsets unite. It is likely that their conversations would center around pessimistic topics and strengthen their shared negative beliefs about the world. Instead of investing their time in refining their shared perspective, they will reinforce their shared beliefs that "The world is bad. People cannot be trusted. People are greedy and deceptive." They are convinced that as children grow up, they escape their responsibilities and neglect their parents. Relatives never stand in support, especially during challenging times, and it is necessary to be astute and opportunistic to survive, as no one is inherently noble or trustworthy.

Their pen drive, i.e., their shared memory bank, is saturated with similar ideologies and a grey gloomy picture of the world.

But, in contrast, even if one of the two harbors a positive mindset, there is a possibility of improvement as they act as a counterbalance. The spouse can guide and enlighten the other, uplifting their relationship. As a result, the child will receive an enhanced and better environment during its formative years.

Unfortunately, parents with a pessimistic approach accumulate a repository of mistrust, suffering, and wrong beliefs, which are inadvertently passed on to their children. The child, too, becomes another Pen or Pencil, brimming with more pain, sorrow, disillusionment, disbelief, doubts, and negativity. Hence, parents must cleanse their pain drive – shared perspective – before the arrival of their child.

Think of this life as a mountain. The higher one needs to climb, the lesser the weight one should carry on one's shoulder. A heavier load will make their journey arduous. They will get tired midway. It is wiser to keep the burdens to a bare minimum, be it physical or mental, on the body, the heart, the mind, and in memory.

Your obligations should not encumber the child. Children deserve to be raised in an unburdened environment to be able to amass their own experiences with an open and positive mindset. Just as you get evidence of your thinking, the child may get evidence of their beliefs that the world is full of compassionate and loving people and that life can be lived with joy and simplicity. Refraining from unnecessarily burdening the child with your perceptions will unlock great possibilities for your child's smooth, simple, and delightful journey.

Q: I have yet another scenario. My neighbor is always complaining about their son residing overseas. They repeatedly complain, "We did so much for our son, but when it was time to support and care for us, he left his aging parents and settled abroad."

A: This is a common scene frequently observed and shared. Parents are either swayed by societal trends or, in an attempt to emulate others, encourage their children to seek employment abroad. They raise their expectations of securing higher earnings in foreign currency.

Left to themselves, the children would have been content with their existing jobs and income in their own country. However, in their longing for social recognition and aligning status with others, parents forcefully send children overseas for higher education and careers. Succumbing to these expectations, children choose to study and work abroad and eventually get carried away by the lure of lucrative jobs and lavish lifestyles. As time progresses, the children desire to invite their parents to live with them. However, parents do not wish to leave their homeland because of their attachment to their roots. Parents believe they struggled and invested every hard-earned penny and dedication into building their house. This deep attachment makes it difficult for them to leave their house and the comfort zone of their locality.

The parents' attachment to both, their children, and their local inclinations is an issue in this context. Attachment in the pretext of children appears natural, disguised as affection, which does not seem like a disorder to people. In contrast, it is the cause of great sorrow because attachment is a disorder that binds a person like a restraint and keeps them unhappy.

Parents expect their children to fulfil all their expectations. They expect their children to conform to their norms and preferences and follow their behest. They expect their children to excel academically and accept everything they say willingly. This attachment creates a sense of ownership, where the child is perceived as their personal belonging akin to their possessions. Consequently, this feeling becomes a cause of their worry. Parents become overly possessive and live in perpetual anxiety for the well-being of their children.

Parents should see their own journey through life and their children's journeys as parallel railway tracks. Instead of expecting their children to always follow their preferences, parents should understand that each human being is like a separate train, traveling on their own unique track. While these tracks may run side by side for a time, there comes a point when the paths may diverge in different directions.

Therefore, parents need to understand that their children are on their own unique journey of life, with their individual experiences. As a parent, your rightful duty is to contribute to your child's journey through the right upbringing, instilling higher values and promoting good conduct. But to expect anything beyond that would be far from ideal. Any high expectations can burden the child with guilt for not being able to fulfil their parent's expectations and having to choose a different path. This may leave the parents unhappy for the rest of their life.

Every parent should reflect on whether they have lived their entire life conforming to their parents' norms and directives. And if the child unquestioningly obeys every command, won't they lose originality? They would be mere puppets instead of free human beings. Effective parenting is not making children follow your directives but rather liberating them from your beliefs and the weight of your expectations. Meaningful parenting happens when children have the liberty to gather their own experiences.

Points for reflection

- It is best to change our negative mindset and wrong beliefs with the right understanding and knowledge before the arrival of the child so that they do not influence the child negatively.
- Give love to children, but don't get overly attached to them. Attachment and expectations are disorders that create discontent among parents and hinder their child's development.
- Children have their own independent personalities and a unique journey to embark on. They have not come to life as mere puppets in their parents' hands. Parents need to be their ally, and not ringmasters.
- Children should be raised by liberating them from the beliefs and burden of parents' expectations; otherwise, all the pains and sorrows in the parents' lives will be seen in the children's lives.

PART III

Right Conduct for a Pregnant Woman

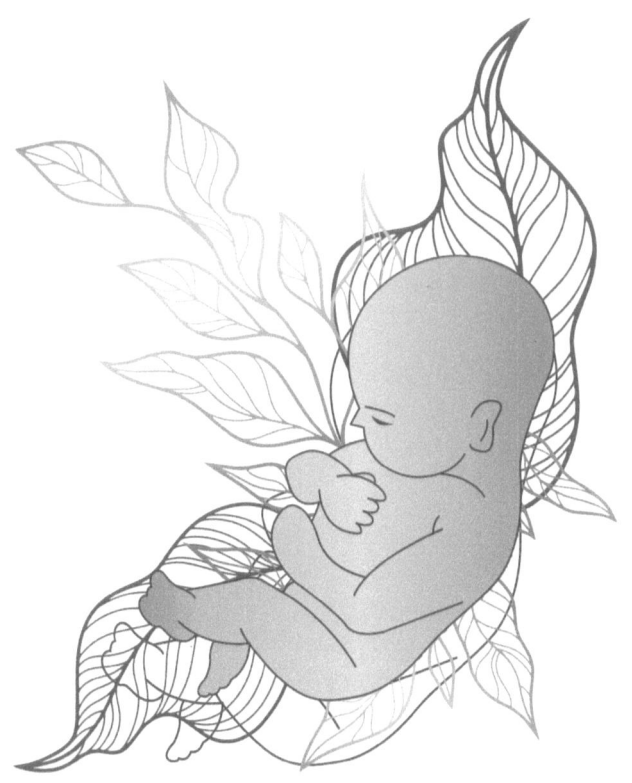

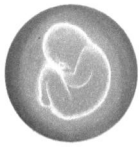

20
Healthy Practices for the Day

With every rising sun, a new opportunity for heightened awareness and enlightenment unfolds. Every new dawn ushers a new day, beckoning us to elevate our consciousness, deepen our understanding, and nurture well-being. It propels us to engage in activities that radiate positivity and dispel darkness. Each morning is a beautiful canvas to paint the hues of our day. After a restful sleep, the mind awakens in a state of serenity, ready to absorb and integrate wisdom, new information, profound insights, and life lessons. This becomes the guiding force of our day, channeling our thoughts, actions, interactions, and behavior.

Q: Generally, people start their day by reading newspapers. With so much violence and negative news being dished out through the media, isn't this a wrong way to start the day?

A: Most newspapers feature news concerning politics, violence, and a plethora of negative information. Consuming so much negativity can deeply impact the mind and create negative perceptions of the world, bringing attention to the undesirable events around us and creating a false belief that the world is no longer a safe place to live.

Harboring such negative feelings is not an ideal way to start your day. This is all the more true, especially during pregnancy, as all this negativity can additionally harm the baby. The baby is an embodiment of pure consciousness that you are inviting into this world. Imagine the impact of such negative programming on the baby. It will inherently develop a lot of resistance and aversion towards the world right from the very beginning. It may even feel reluctant and refuse to be born in this hostile environment. Hence, you need to refrain from all such activities or elements that endorse negativity and avert the transfer of such adverse feelings onto the baby.

Q: Then, what should be the ideal start to the day?

A: Kickstart your mornings with a blissful walk amid nature and perform exercises prescribed by the doctor. This will positively influence the baby's physical growth. Incorporate activities like practicing meditation, *Pranayama* (breathing exercises), reading spiritual literature and inspirational biographies of great leaders, contemplating on them, cultivating a healthy mind and intellect. These endeavors foster joyful and positive thoughts that create enduring and enriching memories for the baby. If you prefer listening, immerse yourself in uplifting tunes of serene bhajans, hymns, mantras, devotional couplets, or spiritual discourses.

Every word or mantra has vibrations. Recognizing the vibrational power of words and mantras, our ancestors have curated various mantras specifically for the prenatal period. Listening to these mantras transmits the highest vibrations to the baby, creating an environment of positivity and spiritual essence.

Envision your body as a temple. During this prenatal phase, you cradle the pristine consciousness within you in the form of an unborn baby in your temple-like body. Consider the example of Mother Mary. She is known as Virgin Mary because she conceived and birthed Jesus in the sublime state of purity and devotion to the Supreme Being. She served as a temple for the birthing of the Son of God.

If you were to offer some flowers in reverence to this pure consciousness, which blossoms would you choose? You would opt for those promoting the baby's physical and mental well-being. The ones that will purify the intellect, elevate consciousness, and instill higher values and virtues. Aim to gather all these flowers in the morning. If it is not possible in the morning, you must seize the opportunity whenever possible during the day.

Q: I have heard a lot about the benefits of meditation and that it keeps the mind calm and positive. I am curious to understand what meditation is and how it works.

A: Meditation has a profound significance, and its essence and benefits surpass one's imagination. As for the peripheral benefits, meditation helps preserve the serenity and focus of the mind, amplifying willpower and productivity. It enhances physical and mental health, ushering positive transformation in life. Meditation possesses an inherent ability and power to attract happiness, peace, prosperity, success, and virtues. However, these are not the core benefits of meditation; these are mere perks. Meditation helps to transform one's existence beyond expectations.

The primary purpose of meditation is to discover our true identity and experience our divine nature. It is the state attained by many yogis and saints. For now, we will not discuss it in much detail. We will begin with small practices.

First, let us understand breath-based meditations. We shall explore some simple breathing meditations that can be easily introduced into the daily routine. Additionally, various popular pranayama practices contribute to calming the mind and promoting good health. These include *Anulom-Vilom, Bhramari*, etc.

Before we delve into the meditation practices, it is essential to understand why most initial meditation techniques primarily focus on the breath. There is an intricate connection between our mind and breath. It is the breath that connects our gross body with the mind. We can observe that our breath becomes shallow and rapid when our mind is disturbed, stressed, tensed, worried, or angry. But when the mind is calm, balanced, and happy, the breath is slow, calm, and deep. The natural rhythm of the breath is disturbed when the mind is upset. However, we can restore the serenity and stability of the mind by regulating the breath.

The prenatal phase often brings mood swings due to hormonal changes in the body. The expectant mother may experience inexplicable anger or irritation, sometimes a sudden burst of tears, and sometimes she may feel elated. These changes in the body can disrupt her sleep cycle and elevate stress. When this happens, instead of succumbing to mood swings, she can restore calmness, and maintain equilibrium by practicing mindful breathing through meditation.

Here is a simple form of breath-based mediation. You just need to count the breaths, and that's it. By counting and focusing on your breath, your mind will move away from distractions and return to the present moment, making you feel better.

- Begin by setting a timer and sitting with your eyes closed for a stipulated time.
- Take a deep breath, and then let it out slowly. This is how one breathing cycle is complete.
- Now, start numbering the breaths. When you inhale and then exhale, count it as one. Count two for the second full breath cycle. Similarly, continue to count the breaths for some time. Doing so will help calm the disturbed mind and bring it back to the present moment.
- Continue doing this and slowly the breath will become balanced. You will experience a deep sense of peace in your thoughts, and the body will become stress-free as it relaxes both the mind and the body
- Slowly open your eyes.

These meditation practices are not confined to the mornings; they can be incorporated at any time of the day or when the mind is restless. Practicing this as a pre-bedtime ritual enhances sleep quality, offering a rejuvenating experience.

Points for reflection

- An expectant mother is advised not to start her day by reading, listening, or watching negative news. Instead, she should engage in uplifting content such as positive talks, spiritual discourses, meditation, contemplation, etc., enriching her and the baby's consciousness.

- A pregnant woman should include regular walks, exercises permitted or prescribed by medical professionals, pranayama, and meditation in her daily routine. These practices promote the physical and mental growth of both the mother and the baby.

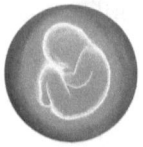

21

Prenatal Nutrition and Wellness

Pregnancy is a gentle phase, and one needs to take extra care during this phase. Gentle because the fetus developing inside the womb is delicate. A grown tree can withstand storms and all kinds of weather, but a young sapling is fragile. It needs the right care, sunlight, nourishment, water, etc., at the right time. Slight negligence can wither or even impair the plant.

Likewise, grown-ups can withstand harsh weather or negligence in food and other adverse conditions. However, the baby in the womb cannot endure all this. Similarly, if a woman stumbles while walking, she can recover from the fall, but such a stumble can harm the delicate life in her womb. Hence, it is necessary to take care of the body in every way possible during pregnancy so that the baby remains safe.

Q: Is taking pills and supplements in pregnancy advisable? I have heard elderly women saying that an expectant mother should not take any medicine or pills during pregnancy. It can be harmful to the baby. She should eat a lot of ghee (clarified butter) and regular white butter for a smooth birthing process and natural delivery. She should consume loads of fruits and eat twice as much whenever she is hungry, one for herself and one for the baby. I wonder, won't she have digestion issues if she eats twice as much? She is also advised to drink milk twice daily. However, some women are allergic to milk, a particular fruit, or other food. They throw up as soon as they drink milk.

A: Whatever medicines are prescribed by the doctors must be taken. There are no side effects from iron, folic acid, calcium, or multivitamin supplements. They physically strengthen the baby and the mother and fulfill their vitamin and mineral needs. Doctors prescribe these supplements only when necessary. Now, as for the diet, it should be decided after analyzing one's body. One should consume food according to their body's natural rhythm and demand.

Q: Please explain this in detail.

A: People typically consume food based on their sensory cues, as if the senses were to say, "Hey, aroma of the food is so good; these samosas (spicy fried turnovers) look so tempting. The noodles are irresistible. Even if my stomach cannot tolerate it, it's okay. I will pop a pill later. Let me relish these." Irrespective of whether it suits their health, people continue to eat and feed the cravings of their taste buds. They often rely on their senses when it comes to their eating habits. But they need to understand that this isn't the right way. There are better ways.

One should eat only when the body demands food; otherwise, the extra food consumed will not be digested. Undigested food remains in the stomach and invites more diseases. The body signals whenever it needs anything. For example, have you observed children scraping lime from walls and eating it? This is because of the deficiency of calcium and minerals in the body. No one tells the child to do so, but the body makes up for the deficiencies by eating such things.

Similarly, when you wake up in the morning, you feel thirsty. This indicates that your body is dehydrated and needs water; hence, you drink water. The body does not demand water by looking at the color or taste of the water. This is a spontaneous process. Animals, too, eat according to their body's demands.

Some people time their meals based on the clock. Their lunch/dinner is aligned to designated hours. They will eat at the specified time, even if they aren't hungry, which is undoubtedly not good for their health.

You must eat only when you are hungry and consume nutritious, easily digestible, and balanced food as much as possible to satisfy your hunger.

Hence, being pregnant does not mean you need to eat double the amount of food. The body will signal if it feels the urge to eat more. Then you need not bother that it is not the right time to eat. When one eats the right food when the body demands, food acts as a medicine that enhances the body's health; otherwise, the body can become a home for diseases.

Q: Is there more dietary information that needs to be known?

A: Yes, there is no better guide than nature. One needs to be aligned with nature and receive its guidance as much as possible. Whether it is Mother Nature or inner nature.

According to Ayurveda, the human body is governed by three *Doshas*. In simple terms, Doshas means the primary principles that govern the psychological and physiological functions of the body. These three doshas are *Vata*, *Pitta*, and *Kapha*. If these three doshas are balanced, the body remains healthy and disease-free. Every human body is dominated by one predominant dosha, based on which we should decide our diet. This is because the food suitable for a person with Kapha dosha need not be ideal for someone with Vata dosha, and vice–versa. You may have observed that one member of the family gets sick by eating a particular fruit, whereas others in the same family can eat that fruit comfortably. Therefore, it is imperative to understand the needs of the body and its predominant dosha and then decide the diet accordingly. If needed, you can consult a dietician.

For example, if drinking milk makes one throw up, it means that milk is not suitable for that person, or it is not getting digested. In that case, one must find alternatives that provide the same nutrition, like yogurt, buttermilk, or anything else.

It is also important to consume food with a sense of joy and gratitude. Praying before meals is given significant importance in most cultures. Collective prayers are offered before meals, followed by offering food to God. In Indian culture, some food is often kept aside and offered to animals like cows, dogs, ants, crows, etc.

There are numerous advantages of this practice. Your feelings are transformed when you pray, rendering purity before meals. As your gratitude and reverence for the food grows, its purity is augmented. Food becomes a sacred offering and nourishes your body, mind, and intellect. All this instills kindness and heightens your awareness and sensitivity towards the living beings around you and growing within you.

Prayers and acts of charity are devotional offerings that make food the best medicine, nourishing the body, mind, and intellect with health and purity. This habit should be included in the daily routine, not just during pregnancy, but embraced throughout one's lifetime.

Q: I haven't done this before, but I will start now. Is there a mantra that can be chanted or a prayer that can be offered before the meals?

A: Expressing your gratitude with just a simple heartfelt "Thank You" is the simplest and shortest form of prayer. Before you begin your meals, thank everyone who contributed to bringing that food to your table.

For example:

> Gratitude to the Creator who created this nature.
> Gratitude to nature that created this food.
> Gratitude to the farmer who toiled hard to cultivate and nurture this food.
> Gratitude to all those who ensured these groceries reached your home.
> Gratitude to those who prepared the food.
> With heartfelt emotions, you can say,
> "I accept this food with respect and gratitude. I have full faith and firmly believe this food will nourish me and my baby's body and mind, making us healthier and pure. This food will give us all the essential nutrients, strength, and energy. Thank you for giving us these qualities. Thank you, Thank You, Thank you!"

In this way, you can make your own food prayer. Regardless of the words you choose what's important are the feelings and intentions that convey gratitude. Along with this, as much as possible, and whenever possible, donate food to those in need. Donation is a way to thank Mother Nature, who abundantly provides everything.

Q: Is there a connection between our food and the unborn baby?

A: Yes indeed. There is a small but effective and important practice that you can follow. While you are about to have your meals, talk to the baby about the food, its appearance, color, nutrients, etc. Tell the baby what you are eating, why, and how it will benefit and nourish you both. Doing this will bring excellent results later. After birth, the baby will eat all kinds of food with great interest without any tantrums during mealtimes. They will develop healthy eating habits.

But to ensure this happens, the mother must eat her food with love and happiness. Here is an added advantage: you will automatically choose healthier food and avoid food that isn't nutritious or could be harmful to your health. You cannot give the baby any information about the non-nutritious food you consume! So, you will naturally make healthier choices.

Points for reflection

- Food supplements and medicines prescribed by the doctor during pregnancy need to be taken.
- The diet, food servings, and mealtimes should be decided by understanding the rhythm and needs of your body and not just hearsay.
- Every body is different, and so are their needs and consumption patterns.
- Adopt the habit of offering food prayer before meals. This will transform the energy of the food into a positive and healthy one.
- Express gratitude to nature by donating food.

- Talk to the baby about the appearance and the nutritional value of the food you intend to consume. By doing this, the baby will develop an interest in nutritious food and healthy eating habits.

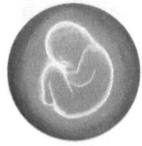

22

Prenatal Clarity: Bridging Tradition and Truth

During pregnancy, everyone around the expectant mother, especially the elders, impose a lot of restrictions on the pregnant mother, limiting her from doing what she wants. Sometimes, in the guise of beliefs, or sometimes under the pretext of precautionary measures, as if it wasn't pregnancy but a critical mission that would fail with the slightest mistake of the expectant mother. Many false prenatal beliefs are prevalent even today, as if it is an unusual and rare event. The validity of such beliefs need to be clarified so that the expectant mother can enjoy her prenatal phase with a relaxed, open, and happy mind.

Q: I have many questions related to prenatal beliefs. The older generation in the household often provides a long list of do's and don'ts during pregnancy. This creates a lot of confusion and I don't know whom to trust. I feel irritated with everyone's constant advice. Please guide me on the right understanding required to adhere to these traditions and beliefs.

For example:

1. There is a common belief that expecting mothers should avoid drinking tea due to its perceived impact on the baby's complexion. This belief is particularly prevalent in countries like India, where there is a strong bias towards having a fair complexion. It is believed that the baby will be dark-skinned if the expectant mother drinks tea. On the other hand, one

should eat tender coconut and drink coconut water, so the baby can have a fairer skin tone. She should stay away from eating black foodstuff like black lentils, black grapes, black pepper, etc.
2. As the months of pregnancy progress, some people start guessing whether it will be a boy or a girl based on the shape of the baby bump. This is quite embarrassing, unpleasant and, at times, irritating for the expecting mother.
3. Doctors recommend brisk walking, which is the best form of exercise. However, others insist that the expecting mother should walk slowly to avoid miscarriage.
4. It is also said that the mom-to-be should not go alone at night; otherwise, she will be possessed by evil spirits. One should not reveal their pregnancy in the first trimester, as people may cast an evil eye. To counter this, she should keep a neem leaf in her mouth whenever she leaves the house.

A: Sure. Since ancient times, pregnancy has been regarded as a delicate phase in some countries, whereas this may not be the case in other regions. Pregnant women live a normal everyday life there. While pregnancy is a normal and happy phase in a woman's life, it is considered a delicate and risky phase due to ignorance and fear. This becomes an issue because everything is imposed under the pretext of traditions without understanding the science behind it. Even if someone questions it, they are silenced, saying, "This has been going on for generations; hence, one shouldn't question it."

The ancestors had created some prenatal beliefs keeping in mind the mother's and baby's safety, physical and mental well-being, and for safeguarding them from negativity. These guidelines were passed over across generations as traditions, aligning them with the needs and values of their respective era. However, with the passage of time, certain beliefs and practices have become redundant, impractical, and may no longer be necessary. They should be replaced with new understanding and new beliefs catering to today's times.

To answer your questions regarding specific beliefs, pregnant women are advised to refrain from drinking tea and coffee because these beverages are not good for their health. Due to the hormonal changes in the body during pregnancy, women often experience a rise in acidity levels. Drinking tea or coffee will only aggravate it further. Hence, without giving the right explanation, a fear of the baby being dark-skinned was deliberately devised to dissuade expectant mothers from drinking tea or coffee, given the bias towards fair complexion. But the actual reason was, and even now is good health.

Walking is considered one of the best exercises to practice during the prenatal period. Moderate exercises, as mentioned before and recommended by doctors, can also be practiced.

As to eating or keeping neem leaves in the mouth while going out, neem leaves have antibacterial properties and protect the body from infection. This might have most likely been the science behind it.

Today, several new norms have been added, like wearing a mask whenever you go out, sanitizing the entire surroundings and the house, washing hands thoroughly, and so on. You need to understand that this was the demand during the pandemic, and rational people will assert that adhering to these guidelines is the right thing to do.

But now, the pandemic is over. The advent of powerful medicines has put an end to it. Thus, making these precautions a tradition seems unnecessary. There is no point in being so rigid about adhering to these norms as the threat has subsided. Excessive precaution can weaken immunity, reducing the body's ability to combat diseases.

Regarding restrictions on going out at night, you need to understand that in earlier times, there was no electricity; hence, pregnant women were not allowed to venture out after dusk. There were no streetlights, and their primary concern was the fear of stumbling in the dark and falling. But today, one can go anywhere anytime as long as there is enough light and visibility.

Another tradition states that a pregnant woman should wear her husband's slippers, not hers, for ease during birthing. This tradition might have originated to refrain pregnant women from wearing high-heeled sandals like the ones women typically wear these days. Wearing flat slippers, slip-ons, or floaters like those worn by men is advised for ease and comfort during the prenatal period. But over time, instead of "Slippers like those worn by the husband," became "Husband's slippers." Suppose someone follows it as a traditional ritual instead of understanding the rationale, and if the husband's slippers are large, it poses an increased risk of the woman tripping over, which could result in a significant loss for her.

Let us understand how beliefs change with time, leaving their true essence behind. You may have participated in a whispering game. In a whispering game, participants sit in a circle, and the first person begins by whispering a sentence into the ear of the person sitting beside them. The second person is then supposed to convey the same message to the third person. And from the third to the fourth, the sequence continues till the message reaches the last person in the circle. You would have experienced that in this process, the message gets altered by the time it reaches the last person. This is exactly what has happened when traditional prenatal rituals and practices were transitioned through generations. With time, they underwent alterations. The beliefs, which initially served specific purposes, coping with contemporary needs of those times, gradually changed over time, and lost their substantive significance.

Q: Many beliefs about solar and lunar eclipses are also in vogue. The internet and TV create such an atmosphere that it is deemed an entirely unsafe zone for pregnant women during these celestial events. Some believe consuming food and drinks during an eclipse can jeopardize the child's mental growth. Some say that the child's health deteriorates. Is there any such rationale behind such heightened fear associated with eclipses.

A: Solar or lunar eclipses are natural astronomical events. According to science, there is a change in the solar radiation reaching Earth during an eclipse. We are aware that observing the solar rays directly with the naked eye during some eclipses can pose a risk to the eyes. In olden times, houses had open courtyards and kitchens, where people prepared food. All these restrictions were designed to safeguard individuals from potentially harmful radiation during the eclipse. However, people now live in closed apartments and houses. While it is essential to follow the necessary precautions suggested by scientists, there is no need for any undue fear or concern.

The fear is amplified by constant exposure to negative conversations, especially the predictions by astrologers on news channels. They have a far more detrimental effect than the eclipse itself. Those thoughts can potentially cause significant harm. "This is a very inauspicious time. May you be spared from any disasters, and may your children encounter no troubles." Such statements trigger more negativity. By now, you already know the effect of such negative sentiments and thoughts on the womb.

Our ancestors were visionaries. They customized traditions, considering the well-being of the mother and the baby, aiming to bring joy and foster positivity. There are many social gatherings aimed towards nurturing joy and harmony. You may have participated in such social events organized by family or friends so that the expectant mother can divert her attention from her physical and emotional issues and celebrate motherhood. Meanwhile, the baby also feels that its relatives and society are all preparing to welcome it. One such celebration is the baby shower ceremony. Celebrated with great fanfare, a baby shower is an occasion to bless the mom-to-be, shower her with gifts, and signal the prospective baby that they are all eagerly awaiting its arrival.

Similarly, many more rituals are practiced after the baby's birth. The *Mundan Sanskar, Naamkaran,* and *Karnachedan,* are all well-celebrated rituals by family members, relatives, and society in the Hindu tradition. The Mundan Sanskar, also known as Tonsure ceremony, involves shaving off the baby's birth hair. The baby's ears are pierced in the Karnachedan or the Ear-piercing ceremony. According to the science of acupressure, the specific point where the ears are pierced is believed to stimulate intelligence. The Namkaran or Naming ceremony, is a joyous occasion in which the baby's name is officially revealed and shared with the community.

Life seems dull without celebrations. In the earlier days, all these celebrations allowed friends and relatives to gather, organize, and host parties and get-togethers. These opportunities served as a platform to practice religious activities like worship, sacred purification rituals, devotion, express gratitude to God and nature, and offer prayers for the baby's well-being.

Hence, any practice you engage in should be undertaken with the right and comprehensive understanding. Pregnancy is a precious and important phase of life. It is an opportunity to acquire new knowledge, gain experience, and cherish the beautiful and joyous moments of life that come with witnessing another life growing within.

Points for reflection

- Many different rituals, customs, and beliefs regarding pregnancy, pregnant women, and newborn babies are prevalent in our society.
- Every ritual and belief was created in accordance with the needs of the time but they may not necessarily be relevant in today's world or times.
- Understanding the science and foundations of the underlying belief is essential before following any ritual.
- There is no need for any undue fear because the fundamental purpose of every prenatal ritual or belief is to foster safety, health, happiness, and positivity in the expectant mother and her baby. It is better to let go of those rituals or beliefs that instigate fear and anxiety.
- The instructions or guidelines applicable today must be followed, regardless of whether they are part of any belief, tradition, or ritual.

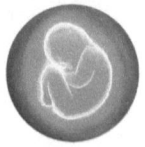

23

Hormones to Harmony

Pregnancy is indeed a time of significant change. A woman undergoes numerous physical and mental changes in her body throughout her pregnancy. While she understands, accepts, and endures these changes, she needs to take a few precautions so that the entire birthing journey is smooth and healthy, ensuring her and her baby's safety. Which precautions to follow and which to skip depends on the expectant mother and her situation.

The expecting parents will have to make decisions based on what suits them using common sense, as what is right for one may not be suitable for the another. For example, as far as possible, pregnant women should avoid long travel journeys. However, if it is unavoidable, other necessary precautions can be taken.

Q: I have understood the dietary habits one needs to practice during pregnancy. Apart from this, what precautions should a pregnant woman take while performing her routine activities?

A: Yes, sure enough, there are some precautions that an expectant mother needs to take during her nine-month pregnancy journey. She needs to be aware and mindful of all her actions.

Here is a helpful list of actions to do, and those to avoid.

Mindful Movements: Be mindful of the physical posture and gait, while walking or moving around. Ensure that the spine remains straight while sitting, avoid sitting cross-legged, or sitting in a posture that will exert undue pressure on her belly. Always turn sideways before getting up from the bed and avoid sitting or getting up with a jerk. Visit the toilet when the urge arises. Avoid suppressing the urge to urinate or defecate and attend to it right away.

Comfortable clothing and footwear: Wear comfortable footwear to maintain good balance and right posture. As far as possible, opt for comfortable cotton clothes and refrain from wearing anything tight or constricting around the belly. For example, avoid wearing heavy sarees, tight jeans, etc. Avoid being in a noisy and chaotic environment as it can harm the baby.

Exercise: Practice breathing in pure, fresh air and practice light pranayama (breath control exercises) as much as possible. This will help distribute oxygen to every cell of the body. Sunbathing in the morning is the best source of vitamin D and is very important as it helps strengthen the bones of the expectant mother and her baby. Do not just sit or adopt a sedentary lifestyle, considering pregnancy a disease. Consult your doctor and perform simple, easy-to-do exercises. Take walks in the morning and evening.

Daily Routine: Continue doing your routine tasks slowly and mindfully. Do not work in haste. Keep the home and surroundings clean to get fresh air and sunlight in the house.

Q: A pregnant woman often experiences mood swings. Sometimes, she gets upset over little things; sometimes, she is elated, and at times feels intense sadness. How should she handle and respond to these fluctuating mood swings?

A: During the prenatal phase, a woman undergoes numerous hormonal changes in her body, which also affects her emotions. At one instance, she might experience moments of delight; at the other, she might feel like crying. At one instance, she might feel utterly frustrated, while she might experience peace and serenity at the other.

These emotional variations can be challenging to navigate. Hence, in such situations, she is advised to accept the emotion as it is and not get carried away with it. She should neither resist nor hold back those emotions. For example, she should cry if she feels like crying and laugh if she feels like laughing.

It is most important to observe and let go of any conflict or turmoil in the mind and body. Do not get entangled in it. Keep yourself active in creative endeavors. By doing this, you will feel happier, and the baby's heart and brain will develop well with creative qualities.

Further, an effective practice to navigate through these emotional upheavals is to share or write down your feelings. This practice will reduce the power of the overwhelming emotions, making you feel lighter. You may share your feelings with your best friend or soulmate. Otherwise, pen down your emotions in a personal diary if you do not wish to share them with anyone.

It is universal and normal to experience mood swings due to hormonal changes in the body. Yet, if you are still struggling to cope with those changes, you can consult your doctor or seek support from a counsellor.

Q: Are there any more ideas that can be practiced?

A: One can practice brain gym exercises. By making use of the hands and fingers, brain gym exercises help keep the left brain and the right brain more active. There are many brain gym exercise videos available on the internet. You can practice any of them.

To sharpen the brain, you can also solve riddles, crosswords, play scrabble, etc. This will foster the baby's brain development as well. Playing board games like chess, ludo, and carrom with the family helps build a healthy bond, and the baby feels part of the family. If possible, read inspirational stories to the baby every morning and night, especially before bedtime. It will help bring purity to the baby's intellect and develop virtues. All these activities will also help in diverting your attention from the emotional flux.

Listen to your favorite music whenever you feel depressed or are in a bad mood. Music is an excellent therapy that calms the mind and uplifts the mood. Listen to soothing light music or devotional songs; avoid loud, noisy music. Pursue your favorite art form or hobby, like music, painting, gardening, reading positive books and biographies.

By pursuing your favorite hobby or engaging in creative work, you need not rely on any external sources to feel happy. You are in harmony with your own self, and this happiness positively touches the baby. Despite all this, if you still feel sad and don't feel like doing anything, call your dearest friend and chat with them for a while. It will clear your mind, and you will feel better.

Points for reflection

- During pregnancy, take special care of your body posture. Pay attention to your posture while sitting, walking, and moving around. Be mindful and attentive while performing routine activities.
- Mood swings due to hormonal changes are universal and normal during pregnancy. Try to accept it without getting disturbed or entangled in it.
- Whenever you feel you cannot cope with the emotional disturbance or upheaval, get help from a doctor, counsellor, or a well-wisher.
- Perform some creative work to keep your body and mind happy and balanced. Play board games like chess with family, solve crosswords or puzzles, and read inspirational autobiographies.

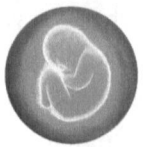

24
Essential Steps Before the Baby Arrives

Successful completion of any task calls for two things before its commencement. The first is a thorough understanding of the task, and the second is adequate preparation before beginning the task. Those, who step into the arena with full preparation, experience a higher success rate than their counterparts.

On the contrary, some say, "Let's start the work first, then we'll see how it unfolds." The primary challenge that people with such a mindset face is fear, anxiety, feelings of despair, and the lack of self-confidence. They are anxious about the uncertainty of the work, its completion within the stipulated timeframe, and its potential success.

The same is true with the birthing process. The various myths and beliefs about delivery instill fears in expectant mothers. As the due date approaches, it is natural for them to feel anxious and nervous. They are consumed by a barrage of questions, such as, "What will happen during the delivery? Will it be a caesarean or normal delivery? How will we manage everything? What if there are unexpected complications? What if I start getting contractions suddenly? Will we be able to make it to the hospital on time? What if the delivery occurs en route before reaching the hospital? How will we handle it all?"

This relentless stream of questions can cause fear and mayhem, and sometimes even provoke a panic attack.

Q: The internet is chockful of articles on the birthing process. People often turn to these resources to gain more information and boost their confidence, but sadly, seeking such reassurance usually backfires. This is because some articles focus on complex delivery cases, and worst-case scenarios, instigating panic in the reader's mind. They begin contemplating the likelihood of experiencing those scenarios themselves.

A: That's right. Browse the internet about your city's escalating air pollution levels and their adverse effects, and you will feel apprehensive about breathing. Every breath will feel increasingly toxic.

Likewise, paracetamol or acetaminophen, well regarded as a safe medicine for fever or pain, is often taken without a prescription. However, if you browse online about its potential side effects, you will be convinced that it is the most unsafe medicine. This isn't to scare you but to emphasize the fact that people express their opinions on online platforms. Not all information on such platforms is accurate and applicable to your situation. One needs to exercise discretion while consuming such online content. An average person does not need to delve into such extensive details that a doctor may need about the human body. Excessive information can be counterproductive.

Although childbirth is complex and challenging, medical facilities are adept now. A healthy body also accounts for the preparation of a smooth and successful delivery. One should not read such articles that trigger fear or panic. Instead, one can use the Law of Average theory to calm oneself. Here's an example: "Out of 1000 expectant mothers, even if one experienced complications during her delivery, there were 999 other mothers who had a smooth and successful delivery, and I belong to those 999 smooth and successful delivery cases."

Q: Yet, the cloud of anxiety around childbirth continues to weigh heavily on women?

A: Being anxious to some extent is normal, but if it is beyond, it suggests that the necessary groundwork for childbirth is yet to be completed.

Groundwork, as in preparing for the impending due date, must be undertaken well in advance before delivery arrives. This preparation should cover three key aspects: the physical level, i.e., the body, the mental readiness, and the necessary resources. Once these preparations are done, excitement and confidence will erase all lingering fear and anxiety.

Q: What does this preparedness account for?

A: At the physical level, it accounts for the readiness of the body, ensuring that the body is fit, active, and prepped for delivery, nourishing the body with vital nutrients like calcium, iron, vitamins, and minerals to prepare it for delivery.

Mental preparation necessitates shielding the mind from unnecessary panic and preparing it for childbirth. Maintain a state of confidence, positivity, and a state where there is no fear, anxiety, tension, or bias about childbirth. There is excitement and eagerness for that most awaited moment when you will see and hold your baby for the first time.

Think of resource prep as building your launchpad and gathering all the necessary things before delivery. Get acquainted with all the important information needed for the delivery process and postpartum period. Formulate plans to defuse the labor-day jitters so all can stay calm when the expectant mother goes into labor. For example, prepare two bags, one for the mother and one for the baby, and keep them handy about 15 days before the due date specified by the doctor. These bags should contain all the daily essentials that the mother and the baby would need during their stay at the hospital.

To begin with, prepare a comprehensive list of all the essentials and organize the bag accordingly. For example, the bag would contain gowns, a pair of slippers, socks, a bed cover, a toothbrush, toothpaste, etc., all the daily necessities. Likewise, the baby's bag will include everything from baby clothes, beanies, mittens, socks, baby oil, baby nappies, baby cream, diapers, shawls, sheets, wet wipes, etc.

Selecting the right hospital is yet another important consideration which ideally needs to be done during the initial phase of pregnancy. It is like choosing your best birthing dream team. Opting for the nearest hospital is better to avoid a marathon commute during contractions. If possible, schedule a quick tour beforehand to ensure the hospital is well equipped with all the necessary facilities, and have a prior discussion with the doctor. Prepare a folder with all the essential documents, including identity cards and medical records like ultrasound reports, X-rays, test reports, etc., that would be required at the hospital.

Another important aspect is medical insurance. While pregnancy or childbirth is medically covered, getting oneself acquainted with all the inclusions in the plan is better. Discuss every detail about the plan to know the health services covered. Most importantly, confirm whether the plan automatically includes the newborn baby. If not, familiarize yourself with the procedures for including the little one in the plan. This will ensure financial security and hassle-free transition as you welcome your bundle of joy.

Next is the birth certificate, generated after the baby is born. Familiarize yourself with the procedure and the required documents to breeze through the formalities without any final-hour rush.

In addition, some important arrangements would be required at home for the baby's arrival. For example, a baby crib, designated storage space or a cupboard to keep the baby's clothes, diapers, a mosquito net, a baby tub, etc. Stock up on baby essentials like nappies, clothes, bath accessories, and more. Organizing these in their designated areas will make it convenient for all after returning from the hospital with the baby.

Stock up all the groceries and essentials for a month to avoid any rush against the clock. Hence, preparing when there is ample time in hand is advisable. As far as possible, enlist family members or friends to create a support system or network. These could also include hiring assistance or nannies from agencies. Ensure that the elderly members of the family, like the mother and mother-in-law, are not burdened with additional household responsibilities, as their primary focus will be on caring for the baby and mother. This period will demand a change in their sleep routines, disrupting their sleep cycle. They will not be able to manage both responsibilities simultaneously. Hence, it is rightly said – precaution (preparation) is better than cure (firefighting).

Points for reflection

- One should not read articles and information that induce fear and panic about delivery. It is better to consult a doctor or a knowledgeable person in case of any doubt.
- Preparations are necessary before the due date to avoid last-minute tension or chaos.
- Selecting the right hospital is another important consideration that needs to be made before the due date. Making a list and shopping for all the essentials for the mother, baby, and household is important. This will streamline the transition when they return from the hospital.
- At the time of delivery and after returning home, it is important to arrange for a support system or hire assistance wherever needed. Stocking up on groceries and other essential items well in advance is a wise strategy to make it convenient for everyone involved.

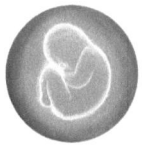

25
Preparing Your Mind for Childbirth – 1

One of the most important aspects of preparing for childbirth is the mental readiness of the expectant mother and her family. Imagine the mind like a constantly chirping bird. This constant chirping of the mind significantly impacts the expectant mother's physical and mental well-being. Whether this chirping is by any family member or the lady herself, it has a similar effect, which can be positive and negative. Hence, she needs to train the mind to consciously think and speak well for good outcomes.

The previous chapter emphasized proactive measures to be taken before childbirth, like arranging all the resources, collating the necessary information, etc. If you adhere to those guidelines, you can avoid last-minute anxiety to a great extent. However, the ever-chirping mind cannot be trusted; it can cause panic over anything.

In this chapter, we will delve into the various tools and techniques that will assist in preparing and controlling the mind before delivery, especially if nervousness sets in or negative thoughts arise.

Q: Pregnant women are often very positive and generally do not have negative thoughts regarding childbirth. But sometimes, people around them share unsettling stories that agitate them. Someone shared recently, "A friend of mine was going to the hospital for her delivery, and they got stuck in traffic. Midway, she started getting severe contractions. In another incident, there was a shortage of rooms in the

hospital, creating a lot of panic. In yet another incident, the doctor made a mistake due to negligence during childbirth." Listening to such disturbing narratives, one often feels anxious that similar scenarios might occur with them. How should we deal with such people when we meet them?

A: Nowadays, it is a pervasive tendency that out of 100 good things, people tend to fixate on the one bad apple and keep lamenting over it. They fail to realize that by incessantly repeating negative stories and focusing on them, they inadvertently invite more of them. If you look at a particular time frame, doctors would have seamlessly conducted multiple deliveries. But people aren't aware or are not even talking about those successful deliveries. The focus is more on the complicated or unsuccessful ones, the ratio of which is very low. Hence, it is prudent to maintain a safe distance from such people. Try to stay away from them using some pretext or subtly steer conversations towards a more positive outlook.

Q: Are there any techniques to remove fear and doubts formed in the mind?

A: Yes, some practices help remove fear and doubts from the mind. These methods can be adopted, even if there is no fear, so that there is no possibility of fear setting in and the mind always remains positive. Let's learn three such collaborative methods. These methods can be incorporated at your comfort, convenience, and time.

1. **Music Therapy:** It is the easiest method which involves listening to good music. But what kind of music would qualify as good music here? Music that eliminates all types of fear, uncertainties, doubts, and worries. Music that instills faith in yourself and God, the assurance that everything will be fine. Divine, devotional music or prayer which aligns you with the supreme consciousness.
   It is good to listen to chants, mantras, bhajans, prayers, spiritual discourses, couplets, etc., related to whatever form of God, Creator, or Higher power you have faith in.

You can sing, hum, or listen to bhajans and prayers or any devotional music that attunes your feelings. By doing this, you will notice that the mind is getting calmer, regaining its lost rhythm and the faith that God is always with us and will set everything right.

2. **Receiving Divine Light:** This is a very effective method. In this method, you visualize the Creator, pure consciousness, or God's divine grace being showered on you. You envision healing and blessings being showered through white shining rays. Whenever the mind becomes edgy, sit with closed eyes and imagine this divine white light enveloping you.

   Imagine the divine rays showering like rain on you, bringing divine protection, health, and blessings. The divine rays are nourishing you and the baby completely. Every cell of your body, including the baby is receiving this divine white light. While you both receive these rays, your awareness is rising, and all the negativity, anxiety, and restlessness is fading. You both are being sheltered in this divine grace, receiving complete health and positivity from the Creator with that armor of light. Every cell of the body is thanking God for these blessings – Thank You, Thank You, Thank You!

   God's grace is incessantly being showered on all. We have to be the receivers. As soon as we become the receivers, we will be able to receive these blessings and see their effect in our lives.

3. **Autosuggestion:** This method involves giving self-suggestions to the subconscious mind. Autosuggestion means verbalizing your wishes and affirming them to yourself. By verbalizing your thoughts and affirming them repeatedly, gradually, these thoughts impregnate the subconscious mind. The information that reaches the subconscious mind becomes the voice of faith, thus manifesting in life. The autosuggestion that goes directly into the subconscious mind comes forth as reality.

For example, if a person is unwell and repeatedly says aloud to himself, "Day by day, in every way, I am getting better and better," then this belief will go deep into their subconscious mind, and their health will improve. On the contrary, if a healthy person repeatedly affirms, "I am not feeling well; something is wrong," their health starts deteriorating after some time. That's why our ancestors said, "Whatever you speak, speak thoughtfully." Hence, never repeat negative words because whatever you say, the subconscious mind latches on to it and brings it into reality.

Autosuggestions can be given anytime and for anything such as health, success, prosperity, good relations, virtues, healthy habits, etc. You can attract good health, virtues, and healthy habits by giving autosuggestions to yourself and the baby.

These autosuggestions can also be given for safe and smooth childbirth. You can say–

"God, who takes care of all the living beings in the world, also cares for me and my baby. We both are safe under the divine protection of God."

"Both, me and my baby, are the children of God. Bad incidents can never touch us; only love and joy can touch us."

"My child is divine and is completely safe in the divine shield of God. My baby is being born into this world as a blessing of love and joy and receiving all the support necessary for their expression. Its birthing will happen smoothly and safely."

In this way, you can convey positive autosuggestions to the subconscious mind of both, yourself and your baby. This will remove all the feelings of insecurity, fears, and apprehensions regarding delivery.

Whatever negative emotions hold you back, break them by reinforcing positive autosuggestions with unwavering faith and determination. It will ultimately end the negative feeling.

The next chapter will dive into the fourth method to control the constant chirping of the mind.

Points for reflection

- Consciously shift the mind's focus away from the negative thoughts related to childbirth and steer it towards positive thinking.
- It is necessary to teach the mind to think positively, as everything that the mind repeats with intensity gets fed into the subconscious mind. It bears the full possibility of becoming one's reality.
- By giving the right direction to the mind, you not only redirect it from negative thoughts but also make it a catalyst for positive results in your life, such as safe childbirth, health, success, prosperity, virtue, and so on.
- Methods like music therapy, receiving divine light, and giving autosuggestions can be used to eliminate fears and negative thoughts.

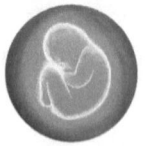

26
Preparing Your Mind for Childbirth – 2

Q: What is the fourth method to prepare the mind for childbirth?

A: The fourth method is visualization. Visualization involves forming a mental picture of an event or process in the mind's eye. Just as you revisit a past event in your mind's eye or picture the future; similarly, you can, in the mind's eye, envision a desired picture or a process unfolding flawlessly, efficiently, and successfully.

Similar to autosuggestion, where you give instructions to the subconscious mind by verbalizing them, in visualization, you accomplish this through imaginary visuals. This process involves mentally rehearsing and vividly visualizing the desired outcomes of the future, effectively communicating them to the subconscious mind. And the subconscious mind transforms them into reality by believing them to be true.

Many successful people make use of this technique. Before starting any important work, they mentally rehearse the whole process in their mind's eye. For example, they visualize that they are happily going to their workplace, reaching there on time, and all the work is happening as planned and in their favor. It is very smooth and easy, and everyone is cooperating. The work is completed successfully, and they return happily with a positive outcome. Such visualization before starting a new project or a client meeting ensures success.

You can use this technique for childbirth as well. The whole family can make use of this technique to ensure safe and smooth birthing. They can visualize that they are happily going to the hospital. All the arrangements are being made, and all required facilities are available on time. Doctors and nurses are all very compassionate and care for the mother and baby. A safe, smooth, normal delivery has taken place, and a healthy, divine baby is born. The mother and the baby are healthy and happy and have returned home safely.

You consciously show a positive picture to the subconscious mind. Else, an opposite fearful image is often formed in the brain. For example, what if the vehicle breaks down? What if there are no beds available in the hospital? What if there is a traffic jam? What if there are complications in the delivery, etc.? All these ifs and what-ifs paint a negative picture of conflict and confusion, manifesting in reality. And then you say, "I knew something like this would happen; such things always happen with me." If only you understood that it was the manifestation of your imagination! Hence, it is imperative to start applying these methods today to give the right direction to the subconscious mind through autosuggestions and visualizations. Have faith in yourself and God. Everything will be fine, and there is nothing to fear.

Q: How do we redirect our mind from wandering, and avoid dwelling on negative imagery?

A: The mind wanders only when you allow it to dwell in the past or the future. It does not want to stay in the present. The mind that can live in the present is the most balanced because our life is happening here and now. We are neither in the past nor the future. Our life is in this very moment, in the present.

If the mind is focused in the present moment, it will give its 100%. Such a mind has immense power and energy; all work is done with this brimming energy and efficiency. Otherwise, over half the energy is wasted reminiscing over the past or worrying about the future.

Here's a meditation technique that can transform your life into meditation. You can meditate while performing all your daily activities like walking, getting up and sitting, etc.

This meditation will positively impact the baby as well. It will act as a catalyst for you to become meditative, and the baby, too, will receive the values of meditation. In this technique, you will learn to stay in the present. The more you stay in the present, the more worry-free you will be and perform all your tasks with utmost efficiency and energy. Besides, meditation will also be beneficial while raising the child, because, later, when the baby grows, there is a greater need for discipline and patience and staying worry-free, which is achieved only through meditation.

Q: Wow! How do we practice this meditation?

A: Meditators and yogis take support of the sound "Om" for meditation. In this meditation, we will take the help of our navel. The "navel" is the point of contact, the part that connects the baby to its mother through the umbilical cord. When the baby is in the womb, the mother's attention repeatedly goes towards the womb, i.e., the belly. She feels the movements there, giving her the feeling that her baby is there.

During this meditation, you need to focus on the navel, neither inside nor outside, but on the navel. What happens every time you breathe? The belly rises when you inhale and goes down when you exhale. Focusing on the navel, you can feel this up-and-down movement. This meditation will help you to stay in the present, and the effect of this effort will be felt by the baby attached to the navel through the umbilical cord. Let us understand it one step at a time.

1. First, you need to set a fixed time to meditate. You may use a timer for this purpose. Then, sit for meditation in a comfortable posture with minimal movement in the body. Feel the activity happening around the belly as you breathe. Keeping all the attention focused on the navel, feel the breath coming and going from the belly. Practice this with complete awareness.
2. The mind will wander in between; sometimes, you may feel some sensations on the body, and sometimes, thoughts may distract you. But do not worry or get agitated; bring

your focus back to your naval, and continue to meditate with a smile. If the mind gets entangled in distractions, just smile and continue the meditation once you catch the mind wandering.
3. Bring your attention back to the naval and relax. There is no need to be tense or feel any pressure. You will gradually learn to live in the present by relaxing your mind.
4. Initially, you must sit down and practice it consciously. Once the mind is accustomed to staying in the present, this meditation can be done even while walking. The more alert you are, the more you will be in the present.
5. This meditation may possibly seem less beneficial in the beginning. But, when you continue practicing it, you will begin to experience miraculous results. You may feel more energetic, tolerant, calm, stable, and happy. Your decision making will improve, and you will be able to perceive things with greater clarity. You will be able to keep any fear, stress, or anxiety at bay.

Q: This sounds great. I have understood the visualization technique and this meditation. I will practice them regularly. But, coming back to childbirth, if the doctor has advised a caesarean delivery, what steps should be taken to prepare for it?

A: This is an important question. In such a scenario, the expectant mother needs to keep herself calm, and accept the situation. She should mentally prepare herself for this procedure. She needs to accept that the caesarean delivery is necessary based on certain medical conditions, considering her and the baby's state and safety in the given situation. It is important that the baby should also be prepared for the procedure.

Q: I never thought about this. How do we prepare the baby?

A: Just as the doctor explains to the expectant mother that whatever is happening is for the betterment of both, herself and her baby, similarly, the mother also needs to talk to the baby to help it understand what is happening.

She may say,

> "My Dear Child,
>
> Whatever is happening is for your good. You don't need to worry or fear anything. The whole family is waiting for you outside. Everyone loves you and will take great care of you. You are fully safe. All the doctors and nurses will ensure your safe arrival. Once outside, you will find a warm and nourishing environment. This will be a unique, wonderful, and pleasant experience for both of us. We both are co-creators in this process."

In this way, you can talk to the baby and convey this message, transmitting positive feelings of love and assurance.

Points for reflection

- Visualization techniques can be adopted whenever you feel fearful or anxious about childbirth.
- A mind that learns to live in the present does not generate thoughts of fear, worry, or anxiety.
- To keep the mind in the present, one must practice Navel meditation regularly.
- If childbirth occurs before time, i.e., through caesarean surgery, you need to talk to the baby and prepare it for its arrival. You will have to convey positive feelings of love and assurance, so that the baby feels safe.

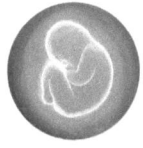

27
The Multifaceted Essence of Motherhood – 1

When a woman gives birth to a child, the child also gives birth to the mother. The relationship between mother and child comes into existence during pregnancy. But as she is called a mother only upon childbirth, it is said that the mother is born with the child. It is paradoxical that the child brings the mother into this world!

Q: I have often heard elders saying that childbirth not only gives birth to a baby, but it is like a new birth for a woman too. Why is it said to be a new birth for a woman? Is it because of the risk of potential death at childbirth?

A: The word "risk" itself has a negative connotation. Life is an ever-flowing journey, and different people perceive its occurrences differently. While some may label it as a part of life, others insist there is risk at every turn of life. Risk or uncertainty prevails even while driving, traveling, or standing. Even the most seemingly harmless act of standing in an open field exhibits life's unpredictability because you never know when a bolt of lightning could strike you all of a sudden.

The point is that you should not get entangled in such negative thoughts or words. Have faith and believe that you are safe and protected by God's tender love and care. The world is advancing through the process of constant creation. Every living being contributes to this progression by bringing forth the next generation into the world through the phenomenon of birth. How can there be a risk in what is natural? The concept of risk itself seems incongruous here.

There must have been some deep understanding when, for the first time, the new birth of a woman was associated with childbirth. With childbirth, a woman brings a new life into this world. On this day, she becomes a mother from a woman, and this mother then adorns various forms while raising her child. In fact, after the birth of her baby, a woman does not take a new birth but nine births, i.e., nine different forms of a mother.

Each form that she adorns is beautiful. It is a wonderful system designed by God, and because of this beautiful arrangement, the next generation receives the right values and principles. If the lady is mindful, this process can start right from conception, for which she needs to liberate herself from all kinds of fears and doubts. If she is unaware, then Mother Nature automatically induces those nine forms within her after her baby is born.

Q: Nine births of motherhood! How is that?

A: Let us understand how she adorns these nine forms. As soon as a woman learns she is pregnant, she takes the first form as *Premaa*, *Prem+Maa*, i.e., Prem = Love, Maa = Mother. A Loving Mother. Premaa means pure, unconditional love. Aren't these feelings born within a woman towards her unborn baby? Without this facet of Premaa, a woman cannot give as much love and attention to her child as a mother does. She attains the zenith of devotion, which is pure unconditional love.

Next, she takes the second form of a *Sankalpani Maa*, where *Sankalp* means determination and perseverance. A Determined Mother. A mother is determined to instill pure intentions and values in her child. Fueled by unconditional love for her unborn child, an expectant mother vows to acquaint herself with the right values and imbibe them into her own life. In this form, she is an embodiment of devotion and determination. Both, devotion and perseverance, are essential qualities for the right upbringing of any child. A consciously aware woman embraces them as soon as she steps into the profound role of motherhood.

The third form that she adorns is that of a *Shravani Maa*. *Shravani* means a receptive listener, the one who listens with receptivity to higher wisdom. The Receptive Mother. In the process of becoming a mother, she becomes a good listener, learns and understands higher values, gives the right upbringing to her child and raises them in the best possible way.

Listening is a very powerful activity. It is a conduit through which knowledge reaches our subconscious mind, transforming into wisdom. Recognizing the importance of listening, our ancestors created beautiful stories. They composed powerful mantras to impart enduring values, timeless principles, and demeanors to the next generation through the art of listening. The very essence of Indian Puranas, mythological stories, and scriptures is to attain righteous knowledge by listening to them. Through listening, conscience and intelligence can be awakened, and people develop a profound understanding of morality, enriching their lives with divine qualities, including discipline, self-respect, honesty, compassion, selflessness, and love. These virtues naturally and easily transition across generations with the timeless practice of tradition for ages.

The stories of courageous devotees like Prahlad, Lord Rama, Lord Krishna, and Dhruva, and Aruni from the Indian mythology inspire and impart higher values to the next generation even today. First, the mother listens to those parables, and then through her, the baby listens to them. Listening to these inspiring scriptures and stories repeatedly, influences their mindset.

Listening is that music that settles within us over time. Hence, Shravani Maa, a receptive listener, is one of the important forms that a woman adorns. A mother should always keep her ears open and receive the goodness and positivity she hears for herself and her baby. In meaningful listening, she also needs to understand what not to listen to. In today's times, where the TV, social media, and the internet are all dominated by negative content, it is important to be vigilant about what a receptive listening mother should not listen to. In this way, along with pregnancy, a woman assumes the form of a good receptive listener.

The remaining six forms of a Mother are explained in the subsequent chapter.

Points for reflection

- After delivery, a woman does not have a second birth, as popularly said, but rather adorns nine forms of a mother. She can take these nine forms at any time during her prenatal journey.
- Of these nine forms of a mother, the first three forms are:
    1. Premaa – the mother, who is an embodiment of unconditional love.
    2. Sankalpani Maa – the mother who resolves and perseveres to instill pure values in her child.
    3. Shravani Maa – the mother who brings about positive changes in herself and the baby through conscious listening to higher wisdom.

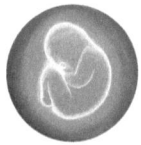

28

The Multifaceted Essence of Motherhood – 2

Q: What are the other forms played by a mother?

A: Yes, let us now understand the rest of the forms.

The fourth form is *Manani Maa, Manan* = Contemplation. A Contemplating Mother, who contemplates and integrates higher wisdom. Contemplation is yet another important activity. Whatever information one receives, whether through listening, reading, or observation, cannot be integrated into one's life unless it is thoroughly contemplated. Without contemplation, i.e., without knowing the actual worth, even diamonds are like mere pieces of coal. It is important to contemplate one's actions; only then does life begin to transform and gain the right direction.

For example, a person binge-watched TV all day and wasted his time. Although he enjoyed watching TV, later, when he turned off the TV, he asked himself, "What have I done today? I haven't done any productive work. What would I have missed if I hadn't watched that series today? What could I have achieved or accomplished if I hadn't watched TV today?"

In this way, he realized the futility of his actions during the day when he contemplated them. This transformed his thoughts – "Instead of wasting my time in such futile pursuits, what other good work can I do that will benefit me?" By contemplating this way, he gave a new direction to his life.

Likewise, mothers who contemplate the opportunity that pregnancy offers, understand that it is an avenue to acquire higher knowledge. It is an opportunity to impart the right values to their children, and proactively steer their lives in the right direction. Mothers who practice this are said to be Contemplating Mothers, *Manani* Maa.

The fifth form is that of a *Sevani Maa, Seva* = Service. A Selflessly Serving Mother. When a woman becomes a mother, she often relegates her personal needs to the paramount needs of her children. Transcending her personal interests, she wholeheartedly and consistently serves her child(ren) without any selfish motive or greed. Because of such selfless dedication, she is considered the epitome of unconditional love and unwavering devotion.

The mother's unparalleled service toward her child(ren) surpasses all others. Her remarkable tolerance gives her the strength to bear every pain and suffering with a smile. Regardless of numerous challenges, she leaves no stone unturned in her child's upbringing. Gradually, this sense of selfless service becomes an integral part of her nature, an enduring quality that remains ingrained within her.

The sixth form is *Santoshi Maa, Santosh* = Contentment. A Contented Mother. Before a woman embarks on the journey of motherhood, she has ambitions, expectations, or dreams about her career, personal life, and so on. However, as soon as she discovers she is expecting, her focus narrows to her unborn baby. She easily makes compromises in her personal life but refuses to compromise on anything when it comes to her child. Thus, the child's arrival becomes the harbinger of contentment in her life. In the process, she learns that true happiness transcends the fulfillment of personal ambitions and blossoms through contentment in selfless service. This profound understanding aligns her feelings, thoughts, words, converging in purposeful actions. It awakens the spirit of selfless service, infusing deep satisfaction in her actions.

The seventh form is *Saakshi Maa – Saakshi* = Witnessing. A Witnessing Mother. Saakshi is the witnessing presence that merely observes whatever is happening in the present moment without being judgmental. Once she conceives, the woman learns to live in the present, witnessing life as it unfolds. She can feel the movements in the womb, understand it, and offer her knowing, compassionate presence to every experience. She sleeps, wakes, moves, and rests as this witnessing presence.

An expecting mother can feel and witness the budding life within her, changing her behavior, actions, and thoughts according to the baby's needs. She knows that pregnancy is a nine-month journey that can neither be reduced nor extended. Hence, she just has to witness whatever unfolds, as it is.

Similarly, when a child is born and grows gradually, the mother's life also blossoms, watching her child's life unfold. She is conscious and can feel her child's presence even during deep sleep or waking, whether inside the womb or outside. Hence, even the slightest cry or utterance of the word "Ma" or "Mom" is enough to wake her from deep sleep.

This state of being present as a witnesser, which she experiences with the arrival of her child, is akin to the ultimate experience of Supreme Consciousness, which a monk, a meditator, or a divine devotee attains. Just as the consciousness of a monk or a devotee constantly dwells in the experience of Supreme Consciousness, similarly a part of the mother's consciousness is continuously focused on and connected to her child. Its awareness and its experience are felt at all times.

When the mother feels the same deep connectedness with the supreme consciousness as she does with her child, her pregnancy can become a gateway to connect with divinity! This also plants the seeds of divine experience and expression within the child-to-be.

Mokshama Maa is the eighth form she plays. This term is coined by combining two words: *Kshama*, forgiveness, and *Moksha*, liberation. The Mother who practices Forgiveness for Liberation. While on her journey of motherhood, a woman learns to forgive and seek forgiveness. When she does not take trivial things to heart, laughs them off, and learns to forgive, she is said to be a Forgiving Mother. The child's arrival makes her compassionate, imparting a valuable lesson of forgiveness.

In this form, Moksha, meaning liberation, is also associated with forgiveness. As explained in the preceding chapters, by forgiving and seeking forgiveness, one releases all their karmic bondages with others, be it the bondage of hatred, regrets, anger, envy, jealousy, and grudges or bondage of love, affection, and attachment. Freedom from all these bondages is liberation. Forgiveness releases the bondages of the mother and sets her free, purifying her mind, and giving her the right understanding of true liberation. Hence, she is said to be a Mokshama Maa.

The ninth form is *Dharma Maa*. *Dharma* = the common underlying essence of all religions. The Pure Conscious Mother. The one who practices the true essence of religion. It is the form in which the mother returns to her true identity beyond the mind and body with the help of motherhood. She connects with the Source that resides within and beyond all beings, also referred to as Supreme Consciousness, Allah, Jesus, Rama, Shiva, Creator, where there is pure love, bliss, and peace.

When all the lessons learned till now in Garbh Sanskar are put into practice, a woman becomes a Pure Conscious Mother. She is the one who practices the essence of true religion and puts all good things into practice, just like Ma Yashoda, who was the mother to Lord Krishna, Queen Kaushalya, the mother of Lord Rama, Mother Mary, the mother of Jesus, or Queen Sumati, the mother of the supreme devotee, Dhruva.

In her perception, an expecting mother believes she is bringing life into this world, teaching, guiding, and nurturing it. However, the reality is the reverse; the baby or the child serves as a catalyst in helping the mother play nine roles, imparting profound wisdom. It serves as a transformative teacher to its mother, developing and fostering growth in unexpected ways.

Today, this world needs a Dharma Maa so that more and more children become divine children. May virtues like love, peace, goodwill, and compassion prevail everywhere. Let there be no longing for any other heaven in any human being; may this earth itself become heaven. This needs to be done by the mother herself by receiving the right pregnancy sacraments.

Points for reflection

The remaining six of the nine facets of motherhood are:

1. Manani Maa – the mother who contemplates with the right understanding and integrates what she learns in her life.
2. Sevani Maa – the mother who keeps the spirit of service alive by serving the child selflessly.
3. Santoshi Maa – the mother who imbibes the quality of contentment.
4. Saakshi Maa – the mother who lives in the present as the witnessing presence in every experience that unfolds in life.
5. Mokshama Maa – the mother who forgives and seeks forgiveness from everyone to clear karmic bondages and opens the path of liberation for herself and her children.
6. Dharma Maa – the mother who understands the essence of true religion and makes pregnancy an opportunity to know one's true self.

PART IV

Answers on Closely Related Topics

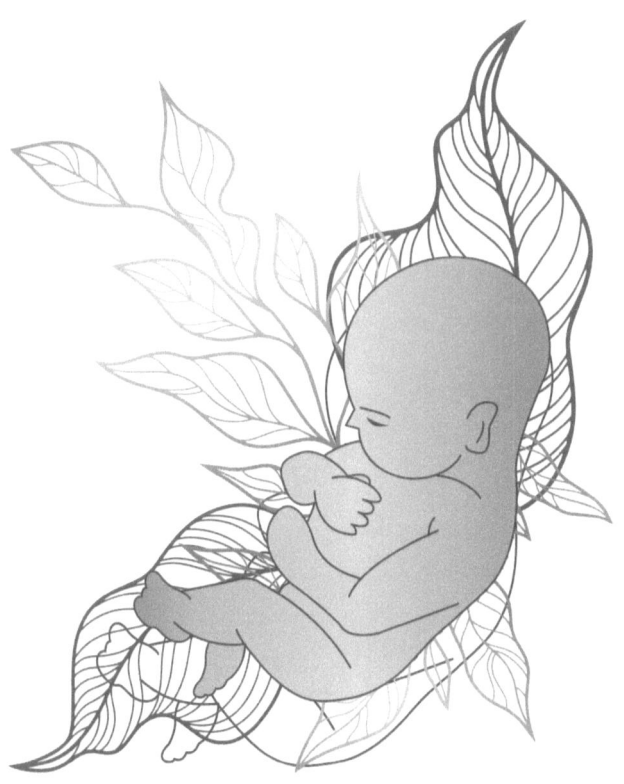

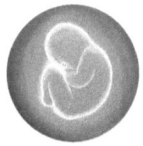

29
Understanding Rebirth and Spiritual Evolution

We are not human beings choosing to undertake a spiritual journey. Rather, we are spiritual beings, who have chosen to embark on this human journey on this visit to Earth. We are gifted with the intricate fabric of the human body-mind for this Earth life. We get to wear this wondrous fabric called the body-mind until it is taken away.

More importantly, our purpose on Earth as we adorn this human fabric is to cleanse and iron out, remove the inner creases that develop during worldly life so that it can be returned in its pristine form, just as we had received it at birth.

As we fulfill our duties as parents, it is our responsibility to educate and train our children to fulfill this purpose of cleansing their body-mind fabric.

Q: While I have heard about reincarnation or rebirth, there are also many who believe that there is no such thing as rebirth. What is the truth?

A: There are a numerous myths and hearsay around rebirth or reincarnation. Let us understand the cosmic play through an analogy and then you can decide for yourself.

Imagine a huge pot. There are different things inside the pot. Now, you place your hand in the pot to feel what is inside. Each finger touches a different thing. One finger touches mud; another touches a flower petal.

A needle pricks the third finger while the fourth finger feels the softness of cotton wool. Each finger gets a different experience.

But who is really deriving all these experiences? Do these experiences belong to the fingers? No. You have placed your hand in the pot to derive all these experiences. While being outside the pot, you receive all the experiences through your fingers.

The fingers in this analogy represent human bodies, the pot represents the world, and the hand outside the pot represents the Universal Self (God, Consciousness). Human beings feel that they are experiencing the various colors of life. But in reality, it is God, present beyond the world, who is experiencing everything. The Self acts through all bodies and also receives the fruit of all actions.

When we understand the standpoint of the Self, rebirth loses its meaning. The Self exists before the body's birth and even after its death. The physical body is like a house. Houses are built, inhabited, and demolished. If one looks at life from the perspective of the house (body), there is construction (birth) and demolition (death). But there is no birth or death for the Self who builds, uses, and destroys the houses.

Q: So, it's a matter of perspective.

A: Yes. Now, returning to the analogy, the experiences gathered through the fingers are stored in a common memory pool. Suppose one finger perishes. Consider that the hand grows another finger inside the pot. The hand outside the pot re-uses the experiences of the perished finger from the memory pool and plants them in the new finger.

In other words, experiences gathered by the Self through all human bodies are available as a pool of memories. The Self re-uses certain memories gathered from one human lifetime by planting them in further bodies.

When these memories play out in the new body, the individual (the finger) cannot relate to them and hence considers them as his or her personal past-life memories. The truth is that all births are of the Self alone, just as all fingers belong to the hand outside the pot.

Q: But why does the Self re-use these memories in new bodies?

A: There are two main purposes for reusing these experiences. One is to heal them, and the other is to bring a progressive evolution.

You will agree that every new generation is more advanced than the previous generation. This is because of the re-use of rich memories by the Self. The world progresses through these evolution and developments by leveraging the rich memories.

You would have heard about child prodigies who demonstrate wondrous skills early in their childhood. You would have seen instances of three-year-olds playing the piano skillfully, and kindergarten children easily solving complex mathematical problems. Scientists are baffled as they cannot explain this rationally.

Someone who is unaware of this game of the Self will assume themselves as the rebirth of a previous human body. The fact is it is just a re-use of memories for human evolution and healing.

Q: Healing of what?

A: As mentioned, the memory pool contains countless memories. Besides rich memories, there are also injured or unfulfilled memories that may have been caused by pain, trauma, fear, or suffering endured through the multitudes of bodies. The Self plants such injured memories in new bodies for healing and to bring completion.

When these injured memories are planted in a body, they get triggered and surface as a reaction to certain situations in life. The pricking experience of the fingers in the hand-and-pot analogy is quite often a result of the injured memories that need healing, just as you need to heal any physical injury.

When we assume that we are separate individuals (individual fingers of the hand in the analogy), we are troubled by the pricking experiences that come our way. We take these memories personally without realizing that the Self has planted them only for their healing and release.

Q: But then, isn't this unfair on these individuals?

A: There is no reason to believe that something unfair is being done by instilling injured memories. Be assured that these memories that emerge within you have been consciously chosen by the Self to be healed just as you would want to heal a physical injury.

If a student training in martial arts is told by their master to tie their dominant right hand and practice only with their weaker left hand, they may find it difficult and unfair or unreasonable. But the master has arranged suitable exercises for them to strengthen their weak and inflexible left hand. So would you say that it is unfair? We understand that this is for the betterment of the student. In the same way, the arrangement of people or situations around you is made for your growth and evolution as a human being.

In fact, more than fair or unfair, it is a cause for celebration! You have received your body exactly as the Self intends. You have been chosen as one of the characters in the cosmic play who would help in human evolution. Nothing is lacking in the body-mind to fulfil its divine plan. Hence, when you accept the memories instilled within you with the attitude, "Thy will is my will. Let Thy will be done," such devotion helps in healing and evolution.

Q: So our role is to heal those pricking experiences.

A: Yes. But again that is just one aspect of the purpose of human birth.

Q: That seems like a huge responsibility and what if we are unable to heal them?

A: The discomfort you experience when these memories get triggered should not be taken as a burden but rather an opportunity.

One might feel stressed, but there is no need to stress yourself over the need to heal your injured memories. If it remains incomplete, the Self continues this process perpetually through new embodiments until it achieves complete healing. Nevertheless, one must make efforts from a relaxed state of mind to achieve healing to the extent possible during their Earth life, as this is one of the important purposes of human life.

The purpose of human life is to:

- Realize who we truly are, beyond the body and mind, beyond the fingers in the analogy.
- Understand the purpose of Earth life beyond the mundane goals of worldly life.
- Develop the conviction that injured memories are not our personal memories. Our body-mind is only the means for healing them.

As long as we remember and are aware of this ultimate purpose of life and strive towards achieving it, we are on the right track.

Q: In all this, what is my responsibility as a parent towards my child(ren)?

A. The first and most important responsibility is to heal your own memories and negative emotions that get triggered. This will minimize the transfer of the impact of such memories or emotional upheavals to the child(ren).

The injured memories can be healed with the help of four tools. These tools are effective, regardless of the kind of injured memories or emotions such as fear, trauma, etc. The proof of the pudding lies in the doing! Hence, practicing them is more important than merely learning about them.

The four powerful tools are: the duster, the spectacles, the cutter, and the torch.

The duster of forgiveness

True forgiveness involves releasing deeply held negative feelings. It empowers us to recognize the pain we suffered and enables us to heal and move on with our lives without letting that pain define us.

The spectacles of detached witnessing

Emotions are like storms raging in the ocean. They come and go. If you are alert and raise your awareness during the storm, you will learn the trick of detaching yourself from the emotions. When we vigilantly witness the emotions from a detached standpoint, it helps de-energize them, leading to their release.

The cutter of "Let go"

Many people find it difficult to let go of things. Such people build a junkyard around them, always thinking they need every little thing, no matter how useless it is – whether they are physical possessions, or past grudges and regrets.

Letting go of whatever we cling to, makes room for something new and fresh, which would, in turn, help the little one to absorb only the best.

The torch of understanding

In the dark, if we mistake a rope for a snake, we will seek a stick to hit the imaginary snake. But what we really need is a torch or flashlight to see the rope as a rope.

The torch of understanding makes it possible to clearly see what we are ailing from and determine the path to freedom. With understanding, we recognize how the world mirrors what lies within us. We correct ourselves within and begin to see changes in the world.

To conclude, by letting go, we accept people and situations just as they are. By seeking forgiveness and forgiving others, we begin to nullify the impact of karmic scars. Thus, with forgiveness, we heal; by letting go, we grow. The daily practice of detached witnessing helps us avoid creating any new karmic scars with those around us.

As we work towards healing these injured memories, we also minimize the transfer of negative emotions and feelings to the unborn. We consciously attempt to minimize the impressions that could be created by holding onto negative emotions triggered due to the injured memories.

Points for reflection

We all are bearing injured memories that need healing. Everyone, including our children, are carrying a different set of injured memories. Each one's stock of memories varies, and it is not clear to us how much we carry. It is best to understand this and start healing them so that we and our children together live a healed and blissful life.

To gain an in-depth understanding of Injured Memories and how to heal them by learning our life lessons, do read the book "Heal Your Memories, Heal Your Life" authored by Sirshree.

You can scan this QR code to order your copy.

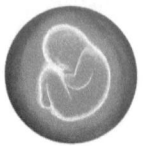

30

Answers on Related Aspects

Q: Is there a predetermined time for a body to be ready for pregnancy, or do we have the choice to decide whether and when we wish to conceive?

A: You always have a choice. The choice to choose the best time can be based on the season, the circumstances at home or family, and the mental state of the couple. You can prepare yourself for conception and maintain a healthy environment. For example, if the couple needs to discuss a critical issue, they should choose the best environment.

But there's more to it. People often pay more attention to external factors before finalizing anything, such as fixing their wedding date. In the process, they tend to overlook the important things that need to be worked upon. People plan their weddings during school vacations so that school-goers in the family can participate. The adults get a break or get the day off from work, and the weather is conducive and pleasant for the wedding. But all these are mere external factors.

The internal work or the mental preparation is more important. What is the mental state of the bride and bridegroom at the time of marriage? Are they financially and emotionally stable? Are they prepared to welcome the change in their life? and so on. Usually, these aspects are not given due consideration, but such mental preparation is of utmost importance, whether marriage or conception.

Q: Some children are short-tempered and violent. No matter how good the environment around them, their violent tendency remains the same. Can this be worked on even before the baby is born?

A: Yes, of course, that is the reason this knowledge is being shared. If the mother develops patience, it will indeed have an impact on the child. However, not every mother gets an environment conducive enough to cultivate patience, nor does she know. Every house has different circumstances. Differences between the mother-in-law and daughter-in-law impact the expectant mother, causing a ripple effect on the baby. Therefore, if the entire family together decides the kind of child they expect in the future, it can be easily worked upon. This will create a solid nurturing environment that will help the child thrive.

Q: In India, reciting specific pregnancy mantras is considered one of the most important activities. What effect do such recitations have on the unborn baby?

A: Mantras, music, poems, bhajans or verses, etc., are the composition of positive words. Words have immense power, creating an impact on the listener. When the mother reads, recites, hums, or sings, her words, statements, and imagination profoundly affect the unborn baby. As words impact adults, likewise, they also create profound impressions on the baby. Therefore, for the convenience of the mother, such mantras are chosen that generate positive vibrations.

Every word has a vibration. Whatever you speak carries a vibration. But you may not feel it that strongly. For example, here's a simple sentence, "Mr. X told me he would meet me tomorrow, but he didn't." This line has a negative vibe, but a mild one. But if this line were to be said in this manner, "Mr. X promised he would meet me tomorrow, but he betrayed me; he never turned up," you can understand that with a slight change of words, this sentence gave rise to such higher negative vibrations.

Unknowingly, people often use such words and add negativity to simple facts. Mr. X did not show up is a fact, but by terming it as betrayal, the person himself gets trapped in the negative vibrations. Such "terming" arises from ignorance; it is the belief system that stems from negative feelings. Suppose this line is said in this way: "Mr. X told me he would meet me, but he never showed up. By doing this, he stabbed me in the back." Just notice how the negative vibration of this sentence has intensified. This implies that even simple words have a specific vibration. And when that word is used in a sentence or a statement, the vibration of the sentence changes accordingly.

With experience, you too will be able to sense the vibrations of words more intensely. Hence, one must choose the right words, be it a normal conversation or chanting mantras. If you consciously choose the right positive words in your daily life, every word can become a mantra.

Q: During pregnancy, women often listen to recorded audios of various mantras. Sometimes they even fall asleep while listening to them. But does this practice help the expectant mother and the unborn baby?

A: You may have experienced that even when you may not understand the meaning of a bhajan or prayer being recited, you still like to listen to it because it carries a specific rhythm and a vibration. Mantras are often used in a similar fashion; even if people may not understand their meaning, they can impact their subconscious mind. The subconscious mind still registers it, even if the conscious mind may not be aware or awake. Thus, listening to recorded mantras is beneficial, as it helps even though you don't understand the words.

Listening to such mantras gives positive vibrations to the baby, which makes the baby feel more at ease and gives a sense of tranquility. The more tranquility the baby feels, the healthier it will be. The effect of negativity on the baby will significantly reduce. Hence, it is necessary to give a serene, peaceful environment when the baby is in the womb. Reiki and external touch can also be given, which can provide some support.

But, the baby receives maximum support only after coming out of the womb. It receives everyone's direct touch. When people hold the baby in their arms and feed it, the baby feels a connection with them. In contrast, only limited support can be given in the womb. In such situations, positive vibrations are helpful. Suppose the baby suddenly feels a jolt from a negative word or emotion; it constricts. Conversely, positive vibrations help in their healthy growth and development.

Q: Does the mother's practice of meditation have an impact on the baby?

A: Yes, of course. With meditation, the mother experiences calmness and feels relaxed. She experiences a deep sense of contentment and her body rejuvenates. With this, she also realizes that "I am not this body." She experiences that her true identity is not defined by what her senses perceive. She develops the conviction that her true nature is beyond the physical body, untouched by the limiting beliefs held in her mind. This clarity and conviction have a resonating effect on the baby's psyche. It sows the seeds of emotional fortitude and spiritual maturity in the child, which can blossom at any time in their life. The deep shifts of spiritual understanding are absorbed by the child and emerge and manifest when they grow up, imbuing them with a divine and virtuous nature.

Q: I have read about Dr. Emoto's water crystal experiment. He experimented on water, showing how different emotions change the crystallization of water. A baby in the womb is also surrounded by water, so does that water become the medium to convey the feelings to the child?

A: The amniotic fluid or, in everyday language, water in the womb is not the only medium that influences the baby's development. Many other factors work in tandem, water being just one of them. Even in daily life, while water is an essential element to maintain good health, it alone does not suffice the need for survival. Rather, it is a part of all the essential nutrients required for survival.

You can enhance the potency of water by giving it or writing positive affirmations on paper and sticking them on the bottle or pot filled with water. For example, you may say or write, "This water is pristine, pure, and healthy. I love you. I am grateful to you." When you start drinking water energized with positive affirmations, the potency of the water increases, making it even healthier for the body. Likewise, as the baby in the womb is surrounded with amniotic fluid, when the mother expresses her love to the baby by placing her hand on the belly, positive transformation occurs there, too.

Q: I have read that children have some inherited tendencies that do not fully manifest in their lives until their youth. However, if, in between, there are any such circumstances that stimulate or activate those tendencies, then they do manifest. But as children lack maturity and are not capable of controlling them, the tendencies become stronger, impacting their lives. Is it true?

A: No such period can be defined, and neither can it be said with certainty that something like this will or won't happen till a specific age. Yes, it is true that a person's health, qualities, weaknesses, tendencies, etc., are inherent in them. But if a person has more virtues, then it is obvious they will manifest more prominently. This underlines the significance of pregnancy sacraments that provide an opportunity for the virtues to unfold and manifest.

For some people, fear becomes more dominant, especially when confronted with situations that trigger their fears. This indicates that fear-based impressions are ingrained in them. Likewise, some people get irritated at the slightest thing, while some get furious even at minor stimuli. All these tendencies are indicative of the impressions ingrained in them, allowing them to manifest and express their inherent nature through their body.

For example, suppose there is a room stocked with water. You can access this room through different doors. It depends on you which door you choose to open. It signifies that everything you need is available; it is merely a matter of making the right choices. Diseases manifest in the body and exert adverse effects only when they receive a conducive environment. But if they do not receive a favorable environment, they remain dormant.

Generally, people attribute the child's behavior to their upbringing because, after prenatal sacraments, parenting plays a pivotal role in molding the child's personality. The qualities instilled during their formative years, whether negative or positive, shape their future life.

Q: I have often seen pregnant ladies talking to their unborn babies in movies and TV shows. Some even discuss negative experiences with their unborn baby. Is it advisable to engage in such communication in real life with the prospective baby? To what extent would it be right to share our troubles with them?

A: It is not advisable to share negative experiences or opinions with the prospective baby as it can have a negative impact on the baby's psyche. If a mother wants to share something about herself with her child, she should say it more positively and constructively. For example, she may say, "Your grandmother or this relative of ours said such a thing to me today that disturbed me. Although there was no reason to feel bad, I did not like what they said. I know their intentions were good. They did not mean any harm."

When you want to share an incident with your child, you should ensure that you share the complete and balanced picture of the incident with all the details and facts, not just your sad interpretation of the story. Adopting this method will not have any negative impact on the baby and will allow the mother to convey her feelings and experiences while maintaining a positive tone. The mother should emphasize positivity in the communication, ensuring a constructive impact on the baby, thus creating a healthy environment.

Q: The feelings transferred to the baby through prenatal impressions later become the foundation of their life. In such a situation, if a child has received any negative feelings, can they be corrected later?

A: Yes, of course. There are many opportunities for improvement in various stages of life, just as there are opportunities for improvement while raising a child. But as we know, it is easier to shape and mold a raw pitcher, than doing so once it solidifies.

Q: How can we deeply internalize the understanding that children have come to experience and express the supreme consciousness? How can we maintain a good connection and a loving bond without getting trapped in attachment towards our children?

A: The concept of a divine child is relevant in this context. The child needs to be raised in an environment that can help awaken the presence of pure consciousness or God. The prerequisite for this awakening is to work on oneself first. When the mother adopts an impersonal or selfless mindset, only then will she be able to impart such values to her child. If her thoughts center around personal satisfaction and happiness, the ability to transfer the virtues of pure consciousness is compromised. For example, in India, mothers generally feel they will be happy only when the son gets married and the daughter-in-law helps with the household chores.

Virtuous impressions can be nurtured only when the mother prepares herself and eventually her child for the experience and expression of pure consciousness.

Q: Is it possible to raise a child who can instigate positive transformation in the lives of people?

A: Yes, it is indeed possible. The more people develop this understanding of raising a child with divine virtues that can bring mass transformation, the more they will help in this endeavor. It would help if you could build a platform within your family. Initiate a discussion with them about your intentions of embarking on an impersonal mission to serve the world by creating a family that will bring positive transformations in the lives of people. Enquire their willingness to share similar intent and support you in such a noble cause, as their support is imperative.

Having developed this understanding, you will attain fulfillment in such work, but would they share the same enthusiasm? The success of this initiative depends on the collective support and alignment of the family. But you need not be discouraged even if you do not receive immediate support. You can embark on this journey with self-commitment by unfolding and exploring your own possibilities.

Q: Please explain lust and desire in the context of marriage.

A: Desire encompasses thoughts for a married life that is full of happiness, where the couple will start a family. All household chores will be done with mutual support, providing mental, social, financial, and physical support to each other, furthering their collective spiritual growth.

Lust is the mere fulfillment of the biological need of the human body. Yet, many people are unable to think beyond this aspect when deciding to get married. If children are conceived solely with an intent to satisfy lust, then it means they have deviated from the very first virtue of conception. Nevertheless, if a couple wishes to change and transform their thinking for the better, there is ample scope for improvement.

It is essential to understand that sexual desire is natural. It is present in all living beings, and humans are no exception. How can something so natural be wrong? Hence, sexual desire should not be seen in the light of triviality.

Sexual desire, which is normal and spontaneous, becomes troublesome when it takes the form of lust, controls your thoughts, and dominates your mind. This can weaken your discretion, and you will violate the limits. As a result, your character, and mental and physical health, will be compromised eventually causing harm to the baby.

Just as overeating, oversleeping, overwork, or lethargy are harmful, in the same way, overindulgence can also be unhealthy. So, avoid extremes, take necessary precautions, seek guidance from your doctor, be comfortable, enjoy every aspect of life.

Q: What needs to be done to bring a change to improve this?

A: To bring this change or improvement, you will need to study all the conditions related to conception comprehensively. You will need to decide the kind of child you aspire for and set the purity of that intention in your mind. When one takes steps with such pure intentions, the result will be as expected. Science has made immense progress; hence, all this is easily possible. Suppose a couple needs to maintain abstinence to fulfill this purpose and is successful in maintaining it, it would mean that they have fulfilled the first sacrament of conception.

Q: It is difficult for a full-time working woman to adhere to Garbh Sanskar despite her willingness to practice them. She feels trapped amidst work pressure, household responsibilities, the challenging demands of time, and so on. All these inevitably give rise to stress. There are moments of frustration where she feels like quitting her job, but the financial challenges deter her decision. Compounding her stress, her unsupportive partner or family worsens the situations. What steps can be taken to alleviate such scenarios?

A: If observed closely, all the knowledge and understanding about prenatal values and sacraments shared here, work only on one's thoughts and feelings. Practicing these does not necessitate the need to stop, sit and take some action or perform any ritual. If only the perspective is changed, then even amidst the busyness of life, one can seamlessly incorporate these pregnancy sacraments into one's routine. Regarding feeling stressed in life, some limiting beliefs at the level of emotions or thoughts are pulling the strings. Even one negative thought is enough to keep you stressed throughout your life.

For example, if someone has anchored a negative thought or a limiting belief, "I am not beautiful," this one thought is enough to keep them constricted all their life. This can instigate frustrations and stress that may affect their relationships. It is necessary to work on the root problem, which is the lack of proper understanding.

For this, one can explore the option of participating in the Magic of Awakening Retreat and dissolve the root problem all at once. Then, whatever the situation outside, one will always feel blissful within.

To know more about the Magic of Awakening Retreat, you may read about the details and benefits in the Appendix section of this book or visit the website www.happythoughts.global.

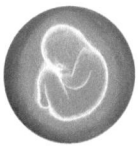

31
ResearchGate Survey and Findings

A comprehensive survey was undertaken to delve into the perspectives and knowledge of expectant mothers regarding prenatal sacraments. Among the 100 pregnant women surveyed, a significant 39% indicated some level of familiarity with Pregnancy Sacraments, also known as Garbh Sanskar. Of these, 39% gleaned their knowledge from maternity literature or elder family members, while the remaining 61% were introduced to the concept for the first time through this survey.

Around 35% of the mothers have expressed their belief in these sacraments and agree with the positive results of the practice. According to their belief, there is an inclusion of different methods of Garbh Sanskar, like chanting (9%), divine music, bhajan hymns (22%), mantra chanting (8%), home cleansing, fire rituals and worship (2%).

Although the above practices constitute only a small part of the pregnancy sacraments and may not necessarily be impactful, as they are not practiced keeping the developing fetus in focus.

About 60% of the mothers did not practice any sacraments. This could be attributed to various factors, including time commitment required for other activities or the inability to connect with the ancient traditions of pregnancy sacraments due to modern-day education or business commitments.

Traditionally, the baby's mental and behavioral development is believed to start in the womb. There is scientific evidence that the pregnancy sacraments and their techniques impact the unborn baby. Studies have proved that the embryo responds to external stimuli. The hormonal secretions activated by the mother's thoughts and her emotional state influence the baby during the prenatal period. Hence, practicing pregnancy sacraments ensures that the mother remains physically healthy and mentally positive, creating positive impressions on the baby.

There are many modern prenatal practices. Some are given below.

Auto-suggestion and Hypnosis

This technique involves imparting positive thoughts to the mind. When these positive thoughts are reinforced repetitively, they have the potential to manifest into reality.

Color Therapy

Color Therapy uses color and light to bring about mental equilibrium. Specific colors have the capacity to elevate the mood and exert a positive influence on the mind.

Aroma Therapy

This therapy uses the olfactory, i.e., the sense of smell, to enhance sensory responses. This therapy also induces a state of serenity in the body and mind. Essential oils and other aromatic elements can be used to facilitate relaxation and de-stress the expectant mother.

Pregnancy guidelines

According to Ayurveda, practicing pregnancy sacraments is one of the best ways to give birth to a healthy child. These are essentially meant for the expectant mother to be physically and mentally fit.

Healthy Eating Habits

Diet is yet another essential component in pregnancy, as the embryo's growth depends on the mother's health and nutrition. According to Ayurveda, a balanced diet, rich in vitamins and minerals, is recommended during pregnancy. Maintaining a balanced wholesome diet and ensuring the right amount of calcium, folic acid, and iron in meals, having freshly prepared sattvic food that is rich in all nutrients aids mental and physical well-being. Further, pregnant women are advised to include a spectrum of all tastes, including sweet, salty, spicy, bitter, and sour, fostering a comprehensive and nutritionally sound dietary regimen.

Light Exercise with Pranayama and Meditation

Light exercise helps increase body flexibility, improve blood circulation, and reduce back pain during pregnancy.

Pranayama, or breathing exercises, offers much-needed relaxation to the body during pregnancy. It also prepares expectant mothers to be able to regulate their breath effectively during labor.

Specific yogic exercises during pregnancy increase the chances of a normal full-term delivery with minimal labor pain.

Meditation is an essential aspect of pregnancy sacrament and benefits the body. It helps de-stress the mind, bringing the mind to a zero state, devoid of thoughts, helping attain immense serenity. It also enhances concentration. In meditation, women feel more connected to their baby by imagining beautiful and positive pictures of the baby. This is an excellent method for fostering the well-being of both the mother and the baby.

Along with these practices, some other activities can be practiced, which include prayer, listening to calm and soothing music, reading spiritual books, etc.

Keeping the mind calm and happy and the body active is essential. All these practices are beneficial for the mother and the baby during the prenatal journey.

∙ ∙ ∙

You can mail your opinion or feedback on this book to: books.feedback@tejgyan.org

About Sirshree

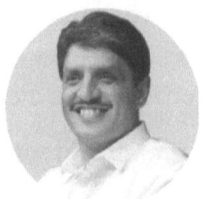

Sirshree's spiritual quest, which began during his childhood, led him on a journey through various schools of philosophy and meditation practices. He studied a wide range of literature on mind science and spirituality. After a long period of deep contemplation on the truth of life, his quest culminated in attaining the ultimate truth.

Sirshree espouses, "All spiritual paths that lead to the truth begin differently but culminate at the same point – Understanding. This understanding is complete in itself. Listening to this understanding is enough to attain the Truth." Over the last two decades, he has dedicated his life to raise mass consciousness.

Sirshree has delivered more than 4000 discourses that throw light on this understanding. He has designed a system for wisdom, which makes it accessible to all. This system has inspired people from all walks of life to progress on their journey of the Truth. Thousands of seekers join in a virtual prayer for World Peace and Global Healing daily at 9:09 am and 9:09 pm.

About Tej Gyan Foundation

Tej Gyan Foundation is a non-profit organization founded on the teachings of Sirshree. The Foundation disseminates Tejgyan – the wisdom that guides one from self-development to Self-realization, leading towards Self-stabilization.

The Foundation's system for imparting wisdom has been assessed by international quality auditors and accredited with the ISO 9001:2015 certification. This wisdom has been presented in a simple, systematic, and practically applicable form that makes it accessible to people from all walks of life, regardless of religion, caste, social strata, country, or belief system.

The Foundation has centers in more than 400 cities and towns across India and other countries. The mission of Tej Gyan Foundation is to create a highly evolved society by leading seekers from negative thoughts to positive thoughts and further, from positive thoughts to Happy thoughts. A 'Happy thought' is the auspicious thought of being free from all thoughts, leading to the state of supreme bliss beyond thoughts.

If you seek such wisdom that leads you beyond mere knowledge, dissolves all problems, frees you from all limiting beliefs, reveals the true nature of divinity, and establishes you in the ultimate truth, then it is time to discover Tejgyan; it is time to rise above the mundane knowledge of words and experience Tejgyan!

The MahaAasmani Magic of Awakening Retreat

Self-development to Self-realization towards Self-stabilization

Do you wish to experience unconditional happiness that is not dependent on any reason? Happiness that is permanent and only increases with time? Do you wish to experience love, peace, self-belief, harmony in relationships, prosperity, and true contentment? Do you wish to progress in all facets of your life, viz. physical, mental, social, financial, and spiritual?

If you seek answers to these questions and are thirsty for the ultimate truth, then you are welcome to participate in the MahaAasmani Magic of Awakening retreat organized by Tej Gyan Foundation. This is the Foundation's flagship retreat based on the teachings of Sirshree.

The purpose of this retreat

The purpose of this retreat is that every human being should:

- Discover the answer to "Who am I" and "Why am I?" through direct experience and be established in ultimate bliss.

- Learn the art of living in the present, free from the burden of the past and the anxiety of the future.

- Acquire practical tools to help quieten the chattering mind and dissolve problems.

- Discover missing links in the practices of Meditation (*Dhyana*), Action (*Karma*), Wisdom (*Gyana*), and Devotion (*Bhakti*).

About Books by Sirshree

Sirshree's published work includes more than 150 book titles, some of which have been translated into more than 10 languages. His literature provides a profound reading on various topics of practical living and unravels the missing links in karma, wisdom, devotion, meditation, and consciousness.

His books have been published by leading publishing houses like Penguin, Hay House, Bloomsbury, Wisdom Tree, Jaico, etc. "The Source" book series, authored by Sirshree, has sold over 10 million copies. Various luminaries and celebrities like His Holiness the Dalai Lama, publishers Mr. Reid Tracy, Ms. Tami Simon and Yoga Master Dr. B. K. S. Iyengar have released Sirshree's books and lauded his work.

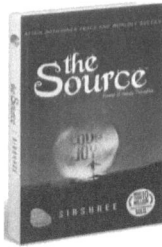 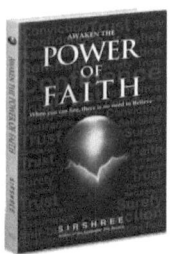

The Source
Attain Both, Inner Peace and Worldly success

Awaken the Power of Faith
Discover the 7 Principles of the Highest Power of the Universe

To order books authored by Sirshree, login to:
www.gethappythoughts.org
For further details, call: +91 9011013210

Tej Gyan Foundation – Contact details

Registered Office:
Happy Thoughts Building, Vikrant Complex, Near Tapovan Mandir, Pimpri, Pune 411017, INDIA. Contact: +91 20-27411240, +91 20-27412576

MaNaN Ashram:
Survey No. 43, Sanas Nagar, Nandoshi Gaon, Kirkatwadi Phata, Off Sinhagad Road, Taluka Haveli, Pune district - 411024, INDIA. Contact: +91 992100 8060.

WORLD PEACE PRAYER

Divine Light of Love, Bliss, and Peace is Showering;

The Golden Light of Higher Consciousness is Rising;

All negativity on Earth is Dissolving;

Everyone is in Peace and Blissfully Shining;

O God, Gratitude for Everything!

Members of Tej Gyan Foundation have been offering this impersonal mass prayer for many years. Those who are happy can offer this prayer. Those feeling low or suffering from illness can receive healing with this prayer.

If you are feeling troubled or sick, please sit to receive the healing effect of this prayer. Visualize that the divine white healing light is being showered on earth through the prayers of thousands and is also reaching you, bringing you peace and good health. You can dwell in this feeling for some time and then offer your gratitude to those offering the prayer.

A Humble Appeal

More than a million peace lovers pray for World Peace and Global Healing every morning and evening at 9:09. Also, a prayer (in Hindi) to elevate consciousness is webcast every day on YouTube at 3:30 pm and 9:00 pm IST. Please participate in this noble endeavor.

www.ingramcontent.com/pod-product-compliance
Lightning Source LLC
LaVergne TN
LVHW041840070526
838199LV00045BA/1367